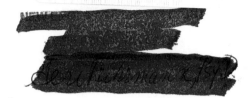

D1037448

LAWS AFFECTING CLINICAL PRACTICE

The LAW AND PUBLIC POLICY: PSYCHOLOGY AND THE SOCIAL SCIENCES series includes books in three domains:

Legal Studies—writings by legal scholars about issues of relevance to psychology and the other social sciences, or that employ social science information to advance the legal analysis;

Social Science Studies—writings by scientists from psychology and the other social sciences about issues of relevance to law and public policy; and

Forensic Studies—writings by psychologists and other mental health scientists and professionals about issues relevant to forensic mental health science and practice.

The series is guided by its editor, Bruce D. Sales, PhD, JD, ScD(*hc*), University of Arizona; and coeditors, Bruce J. Winick, JD, University of Miami; Norman J. Finkel, PhD, Georgetown University; and Valerie P. Hans, PhD, University of Delaware.

* * *

LAWS AFFECTING CLINICAL PRACTICE

Bruce D. Sales
Michael Owen Miller
Susan R. Hall

AMERICAN PSYCHOLOGICAL ASSOCIATION
WASHINGTON, DC

Published by
American Psychological Association
750 First Street, NE
Washington, DC 20002
www.apa.org

To order
APA Order Department
P.O. Box 92984
Washington, DC 20090-2984
Tel: (800) 374-2721; Direct: (202) 336-5510
Fax: (202) 336-5502; TDD/TTY: (202) 336-6123
Online: www.apa.org/books/
E-mail: order@apa.org

In the U.K., Europe, Africa, and the Middle East, copies may be ordered from
American Psychological Association
3 Henrietta Street
Covent Garden, London
WC2E 8LU England

Typeset in Goudy by Stephen D. McDougal, Mechanicsville, MD

Printer: Edwards Brothers, Inc., Ann Arbor, MI
Cover Designer: Berg Design, Albany, NY
Technical/Production Editor: Devon Bourexis

The opinions and statements published are the responsibility of the authors, and such opinions and statements do not necessarily represent the policies of the American Psychological Association.

Library of Congress Cataloging-in-Publication Data

Sales, Bruce Dennis.
    Laws affecting clinical practice / Bruce D. Sales, Michael Owen Miller, and Susan R. Hall.
        p. cm. — (The law and public policy)
    Includes index.
    ISBN 1-59147-256-3
    1. Mental health personnel—Legal status, laws, etc.—United States. 2. Mental health laws—United States. 3. Forensic psychiatry—United States. I. Miller, Michael O., 1952- II. Hall, Susan R. III. Title. IV. Series.

KF2910.P75S25 2005
344.7304'4—dc22   2005000057

British Library Cataloguing-in-Publication Data
A CIP record is available from the British Library.

Printed in the United States of America
First Edition

For Betsy—Bruce D. Sales

I thank my sons, Brendan and Conor, and my wife, Judie, for their patience and love while I worked on this book and other writings in law and psychology.—Michael Owen Miller

With gratitude, I dedicate this book to my coach for his wisdom, inspiration, and guidance and to my husband for his love.—Susan R. Hall

CONTENTS

ACKNOWLEDGMENTS

We thank Nicholas Cummings and Daniel Shuman for their helpful comments on an early version of this book.

LAWS AFFECTING CLINICAL PRACTICE

INTRODUCTION:
HOW TO USE THIS BOOK

Law schools teach about many types of laws (e.g., corporate law, constitutional law, and contract law), but there is no one course or set of courses that teaches about the laws affecting mental health professionals (MHPs) in all stages of their careers and in all aspects of their practice. Most mental health training programs also fail to provide course work on the law that affects mental health practice. Thus, it is completely understandable why most MHPs do not know about or understand many or even most of the laws affecting the operation of a mental health practice and the provision of services to mental health clients.

This state of affairs is both unfortunate and harmful. It is unfortunate because without this knowledge, MHPs may not gain the benefits that the law may provide to them or their clients. It is harmful because it can impair MHPs' ability to meet clients' needs. For example, if a patient is an abused child, a lack of knowledge of the relevant law will impair the MHP's ability to comply with a state mandatory reporting requirement. Legal knowledge can also increase MHPs' capability for handling clients' distress. For example, a client who is undergoing a divorce may have distorted beliefs about what may happen during the legal proceedings. A basic understanding of the relevant law in this area will allow him or her to be more responsive, sensitive, and realistic in providing therapy.

Not knowing the law also is potentially harmful because MHPs run the risk of liability for professional practice that the law designates as inappropriate (e.g., divulging professional information that the law specifies as confidential or not divulging professional information that the law requires the MHP to report to a third party). The latter occurrence may result in liability either through criminal or civil law. A brief example may help underscore this point. If an MHP is asked to evaluate the defendant in a criminal case and then testify in court about the evaluation, the court (the law's term for the judge) is asking him or her to assess and testify about whether that litigant meets some legal standard (e.g., is the criminal defendant competent to stand trial). The court is often not concerned with the litigant's mental health per se, although this may be relevant to the MHP's evaluation of the person. Instead, the court wants to know whether the defendant meets the legal standard as defined by the law. If an MHP does not know the legal standard, he or she is most likely evaluating the person for the wrong goal and providing the court with irrelevant information, at least from the court's point of view. Unfortunately, this has occurred in many cases that we have known personally.

IMPROVING THE ACCESSIBILITY OF LEGAL INFORMATION

Given the need for legal information, why haven't MHPs become more familiar with the law? Part of the reason probably lies in the MHP's concern about his or her ability to understand legal doctrines. Indeed, this is a legitimate worry. An MHP would find it quite confusing to read original legal materials that were *not* collected, organized, and described with him or her as the reader in mind. Lawyers seem to speak their own language, and as already noted, this language or jargon is not taught in most MHP graduate programs. Also, laws are written in terms and phrases that do not always share the common lay definition or usage. Other terms and phrases are not defined at all, are left ambiguous, or are used differently for different legal topics. Furthermore, one may have difficulty understanding whether certain laws apply to him or her because the law does not treat all of the MHP disciplines uniformly nor does it always specify the particular disciplines (e.g., psychology, psychiatry, social work, or counseling) being covered by it.

Legal texts will not be particularly helpful to MHPs or their clients because they are written for lawyers in a language that, as previously noted, MHPs are unlikely to understand and because they do not identify or analyze the legal topics that are of most concern to them professionally. This lack of an organized treatise devoted to MHPs' concerns is a major problem because the law does not come from a single legal forum. Each state enacts its own laws, and wide variation exists in the way a topic is handled across jurisdictions. Multiply this complexity by the more than 100 topics that relate to mental health law practice. In addition, the law within a state does not come from one legal source. Rather, there are five primary sources for it: the state constitution; state legislative enactments (statutes); state agency administrative rules, regulations, decisions, opinions, and orders; rules of court promulgated by the state supreme court; and state court cases that interpret state law as well as occasionally create new law. It is not enough to know about one of these sources of law in an area because the other sources may modify it. Finally, federal law will also affect an MHP's practice and one's clients (U.S. constitutional and statutory law, administrative rules and regulations, and case law). Federal law typically guides cases that are tried in federal courts, sets standards for delivery of services in federal facilities (e.g., Veterans' Administration Hospitals), authorizes direct payments to MHPs for their services to some clients, and sometimes directly modifies state law.

PURPOSE OF THIS BOOK

We have written this book to make MHPs knowledgeable about the laws affecting their clinical practice and more intelligent consumers of legal services. This knowledge is important in an era characterized by professionalization and litigiousness. But this book will not substitute for the advice that one's attorney will provide. Rather, the book provides an accurate and understandable introduction to and survey of the law that affects MHPs' clinical practice.

To accomplish our goal, we identified every legal topic that might affect an MHP's practice, making those that are most important the subject of a chapter, with one exception. Although there are laws affecting business aspects of an MHP's practice (e.g., organization, location, reimbursement by governmental entities, and taxation), we do not cover them in this volume because these topics only indirectly affect the clinical part of one's practice and therefore would fit better in a book devoted to MHPs' business concerns.

And because understandability of the law by nonlawyers has been a problem, we have tried to make each chapter completely understandable to MHPs. For this reason, we have omitted legal citations throughout the text. To find these citations and to understand the specifics of how a particular law operates in a particular state, refer to the *Law & Mental Health Professionals* series volume for that state (published by the American Psychological Association) if it exists, or consult an attorney. We also have defined legal terms as they arise in the text. When the law defines terms, the chapter includes the terms and definitions. However, the law does not always define legal terms or provide detailed guidance to understand how the term or rule is to be interpreted in all situations of relevance to an MHP. This does not mean that the legal words or phrases can be taken lightly or can be replaced with words MHPs prefer. The law sets the rules by which MHPs and their clients must operate. Thus, we tell the reader when such textual ambiguity occurs. Finally, we have tried to help readers by keeping our discussions as brief and as clear as possible.

ORGANIZATION AND CONTENT OF THIS BOOK

The book is organized into two major parts. Part I, which addresses the laws affecting MHPs' business matters and responsibilities, is divided into four chapters covering the following topics:

- license to practice,
- initiation of services,
- maintenance and disclosure of professional information, and
- liabilities for professional activities.

Part II, which addresses the laws affecting MHP services to individuals, families, the state, and workplaces, is divided into 11 chapters covering the following topics:

- competency assessments,
- protection of children,
- education of children,
- marriage dissolution and child custody,
- juvenile offenders who have to appear before the court,
- state interventions and services for individuals with special needs,
- law enforcement,
- pretrial matters in criminal and civil litigation,
- trial matters in criminal and civil litigation,
- posttrial criminal matters, and
- workplace-related services.

In addition, each of the chapters contains numerous subtopics of law. Collectively, these chapters will enable the reader to understand how the law

- controls MHPs' practices (e.g., licensure of MHPs);
- provides benefits to MHPs (e.g., insurance coverage);
- provides practice opportunities for MHPs (e.g., by requiring the courts to seek evaluations of litigants by MHPs in certain types of cases);
- creates obligations that, in turn, create potential risks for civil or criminal liability if MHPs fail to satisfy those obligations

(e.g., the obligation to provide to prospective clients appropriate informed consent for services);

- creates benefits for clients of MHPs, which may support therapeutic goals and services (e.g., laws affecting special education of minors); and
- creates special concerns for clients of MHPs, which may be discussed during professional services (e.g., a client undergoing a divorce).

These lessons will enable the reader to broaden his or her practice and provide more competent services.

I

BUSINESS MATTERS
AFFECTING PRACTICE

INTRODUCTION:
BUSINESS MATTERS
AFFECTING PRACTICE

Many laws offer mental health professionals (MHPs) practice opportunities (see Part II). For example, the law provides that defendants have the right to be competent when standing trial, which creates a practice opportunity for some MHPs to evaluate and testify at trial about defendants who are suspected of being incompetent. Yet, other important laws affect the way MHPs must practice, regardless of the types of service they choose to offer. That is the focus of Part I. For example, most MHPs first need to be licensed by the state before they can practice (see chap. 1). The law then specifies the legal requirements for initiating services (e.g., obtaining informed consent from the client; see chap. 2), and for maintaining and disclosing records and other professional information (see chap. 3). And finally, the law creates formal mechanisms to allow others to sue MHPs if they can be shown to have violated legal and/or professional obligations (see chap. 4). Collectively, these laws address the business of mental health practice. But as noted in the introduction, there are some business matters regulated by the law that we do not cover in this book (e.g., ways of organizing one's business practice). We leave these and other related topics (e.g., taxation issues relevant to one's practice) to a separate volume that should comprehensively provide business information relevant to one's practice.

So why will MHPs need to know the laws that are covered in this section? Consider the following examples:

1. Lewis Jones has been seeing a licensed psychologist and a case manager, who is a master's level social worker, for a year at an outpatient mental health center. He was referred to this agency after being discharged from the local inpatient psychiatric hospital once he was stabilized on antipsychotic medication. Mr. Jones tells the psychologist that he has become suspicious of the records the hospital kept on him and is going to request a copy of them. Will his request be granted? What kind of records does the agency have to keep on Mr. Jones? How long does the agency have to maintain these records after he ceases treatment? Who is legally allowed access to these records? Should the records created by the case manager be treated differently?

2. Mary Chavez was referred by her primary care physician to a mental health clinic because she is feeling depressed and her son is having temper tantrums. If the MHP suggests that he see her and her son for individual treatment, would he need to get informed consent from the boy? Although the boy would become a patient, is he also considered a client? Given the difficulties that Mary has in paying her home bills, what can the clinic do to make sure that they get paid for services rendered?

3. A graduate student has just completed her master's degree in social work. If she obtains a job at a local primary school, can she call herself a social worker, a therapist, or a school counselor? Does she need to fulfill any state licensure or certification requirements to accept the position at the school? Does the law regulate what she will and won't be able to do at the school? If she decides to start her own private practice, what can she call herself and what limits, if any, does state licensure of social workers impose on her practice? If she chooses to work in a hospital, does her state impose any special requirements on administrative and staff privileges? And if she has a supervisor at some point, what are the legal implications of this relationship?

Without understanding the law, answers may not come easily, and if they do, they may be incorrect. These and related issues are addressed in the ensuing chapters in Part I.

1

LEGAL CREDENTIALING AND PRIVILEGES TO PRACTICE

A mental health professional's (MHP) ability to practice is directly controlled by the law. This law, known as credentialing law, is typically organized by discipline (e.g., psychiatrists, psychiatric nurses, psychologists, subdoctoral and unlicensed psychologists, school psychologists, social workers, professional counselors, chemical dependency and substance awareness counselors, school counselors, marriage and family therapists, hypnotists, polygraph examiners, and other unlicensed MHPs). Thus, two MHPs from different disciplines may have different obligations and opportunities because they are licensed under different state laws.

The key concepts and terms that an MHP will need to understand to follow our discussion in this area include licensure and certification; regulation; sunset; hospital, staff, and administrative privileges; and supervisory, supervisee, and supervisory relationship.

- *Licensure* of MHPs theoretically refers to the state's regulation of the title and practice of a discipline, whereas *certification* refers to the state's regulation of just the title of the discipline (e.g., who can use the title of psychologist in that state). In practice, however, certification and licensure laws operate identically, which is why many states now call their credentialing laws licensure instead of certification. Thus, in this chapter we use the term licensure to also include certification laws. Licensure can be described as the process by which a state agency or state board grants temporary, renewable, or permanent permission to eligible professionals to practice in their discipline according to the accepted standards of professional conduct within that discipline.

- *Regulation* refers to the authority of the state agency or state board to control the practice of licensed MHPs, partially through its power to revoke or suspend licenses.
- *Sunset* refers to a law passed by the state legislature that mandates that state agencies or state boards (e.g., licensing boards) will automatically go out of existence after a certain period of time (e.g., 10 years after creation) unless the legislature, after a detailed review of that agency or board, concludes that it should be renewed for another period of time (e.g., 10 more years). The purpose of this review is to force the state legislature to evaluate the need for regulatory programs and to avoid imposing regulations that are not necessary to protect the health, safety, or welfare of the state residents.
- *Hospital, staff,* and *administrative privileges* are a collection of rights given to an MHP by a hospital or other service (e.g., treatment) facility. These rights include the right to admit a patient to the facility, the right to discharge the person from that facility, the right to treat the individual while he or she is in the facility, the right to authorize treatment while the patient is in the facility, and the right to serve in a governing capacity within the facility.
- A *supervisor* is an MHP who oversees the work of another person (the supervisee) and is typically responsible for the junior person's work. The *supervisee* is typically an unlicensed mental health professional or a student in an MHP training program. The *supervisory relationship* refers to the professional interaction and relationship between the supervisor and the supervisee.

LICENSURE OF MENTAL HEALTH PROFESSIONALS

In most states, statutory and administrative law governs each of the licensed mental health professions. This law establishes licensing boards, specifies licensure qualifications and procedures, provides exceptions to licensure, specifies behaviors that violate licensure, and prescribes sanctions (penalties) for violations of the licensing law. In addition, some states have an overarching board that oversees MHPs from all disciplines to standardize practices. The oversight of this omnibus board operates concurrently with the individual disciplinary licensure boards.

In general all of these boards (overarching and discipline specific) operate similarly. This section (a) provides a general outline of how these boards operate, (b) describes the general duties and powers of such boards, (c) details the major requirements for licensure, and (d) explains the regulation process, including the grounds for denial of licensure and for sanctions for violating licensure rules.

How Do Licensure Boards Operate?

A licensure board is the primary administrative body that licenses and regulates MHPs in a specific discipline. It consists of members of the profession it oversees as well as a few citizens at large, all of whom are typically appointed by the state's governor for a period of years.

An MHP's first step is to identify which board governs his or her potential practice. Psychiatrists are governed by a state medical board that generally regulates the practice of medicine without regard to specialty. In other words, there is no separate licensure provision pertaining to the practice of psychiatry. Separate boards may regulate allopathic and osteopathic physicians, although the practical differences in the type and nature of the regulations are small. Psychiatric nurses are usually governed by the state board of nursing that regulates the practice of all nurses without regard to specialty.

Psychologists are generally governed by their own board: the board of psychology or board of psychologist examiners. Other MHPs (e.g., social workers, chemical dependency and substance awareness counselors, marriage and family therapists, professional counselors, and hypnotists) may also be governed by their own specific boards. For example, one state's commission on alcohol and drug abuse regulates the licensure and practice of chemical dependency counselors. If a discipline-specific board does not exist for a specific type of MHP, a state may license those providers under a generic board of behavioral science examiners or may choose not to regulate them by licensure (see the section titled Unlicensed Mental Health Professionals in this chap.).

Certain types of mental health practice are regulated, but not by a licensure board. Rather, another state agency will assume responsibility for such licensure. For example, MHPs who work in a school setting (e.g., school psychologists, school counselors, and school social workers) generally receive their credentials (sometimes called endorsement) from the state department of education. Some states license polygraphers, others allow polygraphic practice under some other license (e.g., licensure as a private investigator), and some states do not require any specific license to engage in polygraphic practice. Thus, in some states one may need two licenses to practice as an MHP and do polygraphy, and in others (although a relatively infrequent event today) one will not need any license.

What Are the Duties of Licensure Boards?

In general, licensure boards have the following duties or powers:

- regulation of the MHP's practice through the granting, denial, revocation, renewal, probation, and suspension of licenses;
- employment of personnel to assist the board in carrying out its duties;
- maintenance of records of its proceedings and provision of reports to the governor when required, maintenance of records of MHPs licensed by the board, maintenance of records of the status of all applicants, and establishment of rules of confidentiality for dissemination of the records;
- establishment of rules concerning fees, forms, and timetables for the licensure process, including the authority to examine the academic and professional credentials of applicants;
- establishment of minimal standards for education and determination of which schools meet those standards, enabling their graduates to be licensed in that state;
- establishment of rules of professional conduct and ethics codes;
- implementation of competence requirements for maintaining licensure (e.g., continuing education credits);
- investigation into complaints of violations, including the ability to initiate the investigation of persons accused or suspected of violating the law, issue subpoenas, administer oaths, and take testimony; and
- issuance of disciplinary sanctions for persons found in violation of the licensure law.

What Are the Requirements for Licensure?

There are four basic requirements that applicants should possess to practice as MHPs. Although there are state variations, licensure laws generally include the following:

- *education*—graduation from a school(s) or program approved by the board or relevant educational or professional organization (e.g., American Medical Association or American Psychological Association);
- *experience*—experience in the field, often shown through successful completion of an approved practicum, internship, residency, or fellowship program;

- *testing of competence*—passing an examination administered by the board; and
- *good character*—possession of physical and mental capability to safely engage in the practice, as well as good moral character, which is generally denoted by the absence of an ethical violation or a conviction for an offense that is specified in the licensure statute.

MHPs who have met these requirements will be granted the license to practice using the regulated title. Returning to our previous example of the recently graduated social work student, if she applied for licensure in her state as a social worker and met the above requirements, she would be able to practice social work in her state using the state designated title (e.g., licensed social worker).

In some cases, temporary permits or limited licenses may be granted for special purposes, and inactive licenses may be issued to persons who are no longer practicing in that state (e.g., temporary retirement or practicing in another state under that state's law). The value of this latter type of license is that it allows the MHP to obtain an active license and return to active practice in that state, typically without going through all of the requirements imposed on first time applicants. In general, licenses must be renewed periodically, which may require nothing more than payment of a fee.

The law does not restrict the activities and services of MHPs who are exempt from the licensure procedures. People who typically will be exempted from the above regulations include (a) registered students in approved schools who are practicing as part of their training program under the supervision of a licensed MHP and, in some states, registered as trainees; (b) MHPs employed by the U.S. government (e.g., in the armed forces, Veterans Administration, or Public Health Service); and (c) MHPs who reside outside the state but who consult with MHPs in the state or come into the state for purposes other than practice (e.g., speaking engagements) or who practice within the state for a limited period of time (e.g., less than 2 weeks).

What Are the Limits on a Mental Health Professional's Practice?

The regulation of practice generally specifies what MHPs can and cannot do. As to what MHPs can do, the law typically defines the permissible scope of practice for licensed MHPs (e.g., conduct psychotherapy and dispense medications). As to what MHPs cannot do, the licensure law will describe the powers of the state agency or state board to investigate and adjudicate violations of the law, specify reasons for sanctioning those found in violation of the law, and list the type of sanctions that the agency or board can impose. Specifically, licenses may be suspended, revoked, or placed on probationary status if the MHP

- procures a license or provides services in a fraudulent or deceitful manner;
- is convicted of a felony or any offense involving moral turpitude (i.e., offenses demonstrating immorality or dishonesty, such as fraud and theft);
- is committed to a mental health treatment agency or is declared legally incompetent;
- habitually abuses alcohol, illegal narcotics, or other disabling drugs;
- is in repeated or willful violation of the licensure law;
- refuses to cooperate with the licensure board; or
- engages in various types of unprofessional conduct or malpractice (e.g., betraying professional confidences or being grossly negligent in practice).

Boards have broad powers to investigate violations of the law. The board may examine and copy any physical evidence and issue subpoenas compelling the testimony of witnesses or the production of documents (e.g., records and charts) in the MHP's possession. This investigation may include the client who brought the issue to the attention of the board, which means that the MHP cannot claim confidentiality (and privilege; see chap. 3) to protect him- or herself from detailed scrutiny. The board may call a hearing if there are reasonable grounds to support the complaint. At the hearing, the MHP has the right to an attorney and to produce and cross-examine witnesses. At the conclusion of the hearing, the board may dismiss the complaint, issue an educational warning, or impose a sanction on the MHP.

Violations of the licensure law may also result in MHPs being criminally or civilly prosecuted. For example, nurses who practice without holding a valid, current license may be found guilty of a misdemeanor in one state. Clients who bring complaints against MHPs before the licensure board may also sue the MHP in civil court (e.g., for malpractice, breach of contract, or breach of warranty; see chap. 4).

UNLICENSED MENTAL HEALTH PROFESSIONALS

Ever wonder why some people appear to practice as MHPs without a license? The answer is relatively straightforward. Some states do not have a licensure requirement, board, or process for some types of MHP disciplines, and even if they do, there are conditions under which the unlicensed MHP may be able to legally practice.

What Title May a Mental Health Professional Use?

As previously discussed, in some states the law regulates mental health practice and the associated professional title by prescribing education, experience, and skills. In these states, MHPs would have to obtain a license to use the desired title. But not all MHP practice titles are always regulated. MHPs may use unregulated titles at their own discretion. For example, some states do not regulate the title *psychotherapist*. Thus, any person regardless of his or her training or experience may use that title. Be careful, however. If one is licensed as an MHP and chooses to advertise him- or herself, that individual should consult the licensure law and the board's regulations to make sure that he or she is using the correct legal title and is not violating any of its rules.

May One Practice as a Subdoctoral or Unlicensed Mental Health Professional?

The minimum educational level for practice is the doctorate for most psychologists and all psychiatrists. But that is not the case for social workers and counselors. States have the power to allow MHPs to practice with whatever level of education the legislature decides is appropriate (e.g., the MSW for social work). But if the doctorate is required for a particular discipline, the issue arises whether subdoctoral, unlicensed persons may practice that profession or discipline. The answer depends on the licensure law in the MHP's state. In some states, the less educated person, who does not qualify for independent practice of a discipline, may practice if supervised by a licensed professional in that discipline. Typically, the unlicensed person would be called an assistant or associate (e.g., psychological assistant). Other states allow these people to practice as MHPs using a different title (e.g., psychotherapist or mental health counselor). This occurs in one of two ways. Either the state licensure law for psychotherapists allows the lower level of education to be used to qualify for licensure or the state does not have a psychotherapist licensure law, and thus, the title is unregulated, which means anyone can use it! Finally, some states allow individuals without the requisite education to practice the discipline (e.g., psychology) if they fit within an express exemption to the licensing law. One example of this is the practitioner who wants to work for a state or federal agency or facility. Typically such employees are exempt from the state's licensure requirements.

How Is a Mental Health Professional Regulated if He or She Doesn't Have a License?

If less educated MHPs are practicing as assistants or associates, they are regulated under the discipline's licensure law. If MHPs are using an unregulated title to practice, then they must look to the law, other than the licensure law, to learn about their obligations and rights. However, there typically is no or very little law regulating unlicensed MHPs' practice. The ones who lose most often in this case are the unlicensed MHPs' clients. For example, to learn about confidentiality of their clients' information, unlicensed MHPs must check the state confidentiality statutes. What clients and practitioners will typically find is that there are no confidentiality rights when going to unlicensed MHPs. Similarly, these MHPs are held to a lower standard of professional practice than licensed MHPs, so clients receive much less protection against malpractice. Unlicensed MHPs also lose out on certain benefits. For example, these MHPs may not be eligible for insurance or other reimbursement.

SUNSET OF CREDENTIALING AGENCIES AND REGULATIONS

The sunset law is the means by which the state legislature reviews and revises most facets of state government, from entire departments to small commissions. The law works by automatically terminating the state agency or board unless the legislature, after a mandatory review of the agency's or board's past work, extends the authorization date for its continued existence. Not all states have sunset laws, and in most states the sunset law does not pertain to the state board of education (which regulates school psychologists, school counselors, etc.) because it operates under the authority of the state constitution.

MHPs should be aware of a sunset law in their state because it creates the possibility for major changes to a profession, including termination of the MHPs' board. Thus, MHPs may want to become involved with their state professional association or licensure board and participate in the legislature's sunset review of the board for their discipline. This review process involves a public hearing that receives testimony concerning the board's relationship with the public, determines whether there is a continuing need to provide licensure of MHPs in their discipline, and determines whether the current board or agency is necessary to oversee that process. The hearing also provides an excellent opportunity to lobby for changes in the existing law.

HOSPITAL, STAFF, AND ADMINISTRATIVE PRIVILEGES

General hospitals and specialized facilities (e.g., mental health institutions) must employ certified and qualified staff to meet the different needs (e.g., psychological, medical, and physical therapy) of their clients. In most states, MHPs are granted the privilege to practice in such facilities. Although the law in many states governs which types of MHPs are eligible for these hospital, staff, and administrative privileges, some states have different laws for general hospitals, public mental health hospitals or institutions, and private mental health facilities.

May a Mental Health Professional Be Granted Staff Privileges?

Staff privileges enable the MHP to have membership on the medical or other titled staff and to practice in a hospital or other mental health facility.

Such practice privileges may permit the MHP to admit patients, treat them, and discharge them from the facility. Although at some facilities only members of the medical staff may have all of these powers, some state laws require that the granting of privileges be done in a nondiscriminatory manner so that physicians are not favored at mental health facilities or units.

Staff privileges are governed by the rules and regulations of the state's department of health, other national accreditation commissions or agencies (e.g., the Joint Commission on the Accreditation of Hospitals), and the institution's rules and bylaws. Such laws and rules also generally cover procedures for the review of denial of staff privileges. Staff privileges may differ by the type of hospital—general, rural, or specialty (e.g., mental health or substance abuse). All three types require that there be an officially recognized staff person or committee responsible for overseeing the granting of staff privileges and the quality of care.

May a Mental Health Professional Hold an Agency or Administrative Position?

State law may also regulate who may serve in certain administrative positions within hospitals or other facilities (e.g., clinical director). In some cases, the state law may exclude some classes of MHPs from these positions. For example, only psychiatrists may qualify for some positions because they are licensed physicians.

SUPERVISORY RELATIONSHIP

Another legally regulated business arrangement that will affect an MHP's clinical services is supervision. During the course of one's career as an MHP, an individual will probably encounter both sides of this relationship, first as a supervisee and later as a supervisor.

What Are a Mental Health Professional's Responsibilities as a Supervisee?

Paraprofessionals, students, and trainees often work with other MHPs who employ or train and supervise them. As previously reviewed in this chapter, state licensure law usually requires such unlicensed persons to be supervised, to meet minimum educational standards, to use the appropriate title, and not to hold themselves out beyond the scope of their practice and competency level. Thus, supervisees should become familiar with their state's relevant licensure law. In addition, supervisees who conduct therapy must inform their clients of confidentiality limits (see chap. 3), including the need to discuss clients' cases with their supervisors. Last, to ensure that their rights are protected, supervisees should also be aware of the laws that affect supervisors.

What Are a Mental Health Professional's Responsibilities as a Supervisor?

Because MHPs can sometimes benefit from employing graduate students and other unlicensed MHPs as low-wage or volunteer assistants, trainees, externs, or interns, state law sets standards for the fair use of such supervisees. To protect supervisees from exploitation and the public from substandard service, the law in many states sets minimum qualifications for supervisors, specifies minimum supervision standards, limits the number of interns that a licensed MHP may supervise, requires interns to be registered, and makes illegal the practice of charging interns for supervision by the licensed MHP. In addition, MHPs may not exploit or sexually harass their supervisees and employees or discriminate against them on the basis of ethnicity or other protected classification recognized by the state.

Because supervising MHPs also have the duty to provide clients with competent services, supervisors should only hire competent employees and give them duties that correspond to supervisees' skills. To facilitate supervisees' growth, supervisors are responsible for providing competent training, including providing regular professional reviews and evaluations of the supervisees' work. In addition, clients during the informed consent process (see chap. 2) should be told that the supervisee who is providing the service will be discussing the case with the supervisor. Finally, to prevent the misuse of psychological testing by supervisees or others, supervisors must monitor the process and the product of their testing (i.e., the report).

2

INITIATING SERVICES

Providing therapy and other mental health services is a business in the eyes of the law. As such, there are economic and contractual components to a mental health professional's (MHP's) relationship with each client as well as with the entities that may pay for or reimburse the MHP for his or her services. For example, when initiating services with clients, an MHP should provide them with sufficient information to allow them to consent to the services. This process, which is known as informed consent, protects both the MHP's interests and those of his or her clients and should be formalized in a signed written document.

The key concepts and terms that an MHP will need to understand to follow the legal discussions in this area include client, patient, "usual, customary, and reasonable" (UCR), and third-party payer.

- A *client*, for legal purposes, is the individual or entity that enters into a contract with the MHP to provide the services for the patient. The client is legally responsible for the payment for mental health services (e.g., such as when the client is the parent and the patient is his or her child) unless the contract for the mental health services specifies otherwise. This might occur, for example, when the client is the court, and it orders the referred patient's estate to pay the MHP. Finally, the client may be the patient, such as when an adult seeks services voluntarily with an MHP.

- A *patient*, for legal purposes, is the recipient of services, although many MHPs refer to patients as their clients.
- A UCR fee refers to a rate that is calculated by insurance companies to determine what an MHP of the same discipline in that geographic area generally charges for services.
- A *third-party payer* is any person or entity that makes payments for services on behalf of the individual receiving treatment. Third-party payers include insurance companies (e.g., Blue Cross and Blue Shield, HMOs, and PPOs), self-insured employers, or governmental programs (e.g., Medicare and Medicaid).

INFORMED CONSENT TO SERVICES

Informed consent basically involves the process of discussions between the MHP and a potential client that leads to an informed choice by the client about whether to initiate services. Informed consent should be obtained prior to the initiation of any services and typically occurs immediately after services are requested. The law is relevant to this process because it provides guidelines for it and addresses what should be discussed during it (e.g., confidentiality conditions and exceptions, such as child abuse reporting; see chap. 3). The failure to obtain informed consent renders one liable to a lawsuit (see chap. 4).

Does Informed Consent Have to Be in Writing?

Whether a written agreement is legally required in an MHP's practice depends on his or her professional discipline, how state law regulates that discipline, and the type of service offered. For example, psychologists and psychiatrists may be mandated to secure written consent under state law, whereas nonlicensed therapists may not be. In addition, written consent may be required for aversive conditioning but not for verbal psychotherapy. Even if not mandated by state law, an MHP should get written consent because the clients may later deny having given oral consent if they choose to sue for any reason.

What Is Involved in Obtaining Informed Consent?

For consent to be legally informed, it must meet three criteria. First, one's client must be *competent* to consent to services. The competency of the client is presumed unless the client is a minor or has a mental disorder that makes it questionable whether he or she can enter into agreements. The fact that a person is seeking mental health services does not make his or her competency suspect. Second, there must be adequate disclosure by the MHP of *information* relevant to the nature and risks of the proposed professional services and any other information that might materially affect the potential client's willingness to enter into services with the MHP. The majority of states require MHPs to disclose to the client all information that a reasonable person would want to know before deciding whether to accept treatment. A minority of states require MHPs to disclose only the information that like practitioners would disclose. Third, the consent must be *voluntarily* given to the MHP by the client. The voluntary requirement refers to whether the consent has been obtained without fraud, coercion, or duress.

During the informed consent process, an MHP should provide information concerning the

- nature of the problem;
- nature and scope of services to be provided;
- approximate length of time of the service;
- benefits, risks, and limits of the service;
- alternative treatments, if any;
- likely results if the client remains untreated;
- fee structure for his or her services (e.g., charges per session);
- policies regarding services (e.g., charges for missed sessions);
- general rule of confidentiality and its exceptions (see chap. 3); and
- client's commitment to paying for the services and agreeing to the MHP's policies.

The scope of the information required can be expanded by the client's instructions. For instance, a client may tell an MHP that he or she wishes to avoid any treatment that might alter some aspect of his or her life (e.g., an action by the MHP that might jeopardize the client's ability to continue in his or her present job). If this occurs, the MHP is under a duty to inform the client of all risks pertaining to the client's concern even though a reasonable MHP would not normally do so. Once the MHP informs the client of the required and requested information, it is up to the client to make the final decision about initiating services.

Finally, it is important to remember that the client is consenting to the MHP's proposed conduct, not to the consequences of the services. The MHP must merely disclose to the client the relative risks of a particular course of services. One does not have to promise a particular outcome. Once the client has consented, he or she cannot later complain that consent was given only on the condition of a successful outcome.

Are There Special Requirements for Obtaining Informed Consent That Are Relevant to Sharing Client Information?

As noted earlier, if an MHP needs to obtain information about the client from other people or organizations or if an MHP needs to share information about the client with other people or organizations (see chap. 3), he or she must obtain the client's informed consent before doing so. For the client's consent to be valid, he or she must receive information about what information is going to be requested or provided, the person who or entity that will be given the information or will receive the information, and the general purpose(s) for which the information will be used. Some states require written consent for such releases of information and may specify not only the form that such a document must take but the procedure for releasing such information.

For example, sometimes one MHP may request that the client sign a consent to release and receive information about the results of psychological testing that had been previously done by another MHP with the client. Some states' licensure laws specifically provide that a client's raw test data or psychometric testing materials may be released only with the client's written consent and only to licensed psychologists designated by the client. In chapter 3, we discuss the law regulating how a client's test data may be released directly to the client, health care decision makers, or to the court.

INFORMED CONSENT TO SERVICES FOR A MINOR

MHPs who offer services to young clients must first determine who, from a legal perspective, is the client—the minor or the parent. State law may or may not address this issue directly. In general, parents and guardians are responsible for providing their children with food, clothing, shelter, and medical and professional care. Thus, they are generally considered to have the right to select the MHP and to receive all relevant information about their children's diagnosis and treatment (especially when they are the ones who pay for the services). Under this logic, which is the prevailing legal rule on the topic, the child is the patient (service recipient) but the parents are the clients (the individuals who pay for and who enter into contract with the MHP to provide the services for the patient). Returning to our example of Mary Chavez (described in the introduction to Part I), if the MHP saw them both individually, Mary would be both the client and a patient, and her son would only be a patient. It is important to obtain consent from the appropriate person before providing services because failure to do so is grounds for a malpractice suit or other type of civil or criminal liability (see chap. 4).

May a Minor Consent to Services?

Whenever a minor requests services without the parents' knowledge or consent, it is essential for the MHP to determine whether the minor has the legal right to consent to the services. Although, as just noted, the general rule is that a minor may not consent to treatment without parental consent for the services, there are exceptions to this rule that vary from state to state. Some states allow minors to be treated without parental consent in emergency situations. Other states have laws that allow *emancipated minors* to consent to medical treatment. For example, one state allows minors to consent to medical treatment if they are married, widowed or divorced, the parent of a child, in the military, pregnant or believed to be, or living apart from parents and managing their own affairs. Last, state law varies as to whether minors are allowed to give consent for treatment for narcotic addiction, treatment for sexually transmitted disease, admission to mental health and alcoholism centers, and abortion (see chap. 5).

When minors are allowed to consent to services, they are both the client and the patient, and their communications with the MHP are confidential and privileged (see chap. 3). This means that any information concerning the treatment cannot be released to the parents without first obtaining the consent of the minor. In our example, if Mary Chavez's son was 16 years old and living in a state that recognized his emancipated minor status, he could consent to treatment and be both patient and client. As a result, Mary would not have access to confidential information about her son's treatment unless her son consented to a release of information. However, this may not hold true in all cases. For example, one state's law permits physicians treating a minor for drug abuse without parental consent to inform parents or guardians about any treatment given or needed regardless of the minor's wishes.

May the Noncustodial Parent Consent to a Minor's Treatment?

An MHP may be asked to provide services to youth at the request of a divorced, noncustodial parent. Noncustodial means that the parent does not have legal custody of the child, although he or she has physical custody at certain times under a court decree (e.g., temporary visitation rights). If MHPs comply with the request of a noncustodial parent for services for the child, would they be liable for malpractice for failing to obtain consent from the custodial parent?

In some states, the parent who has legal custody exercises exclusive authority concerning the care and upbringing of the child and is the only parent who can consent to services. In these states, the noncustodial parent does not have authority to give legal consent for an evaluation or for treatment of the child. Thus, if the MHP does not first obtain permission of the parent with legal custody, he or she is vulnerable to a malpractice claim on the basis that consent to the services was not given. Some states, however, do not apply this rule to emergency situations.

Parents can avoid this dilemma by

- obtaining joint legal custody,
- securing an agreement with the custodial parent that the noncustodial parent is allowed to make decisions when the child is in his or her custody (e.g., during visitation), or
- filing a motion in court alleging that the child's emotional development will be significantly impaired unless the noncustodial parent can have the child provided with MHP services.

Thus, an MHP needs to carefully probe the custodial status of the parent who solicits service for his or her child. Not to do so places the MHP in legal jeopardy. In addition to being vulnerable to a malpractice suit (see chap. 4), state law may also provide that the MHP has committed *custodial interference* if he or she knowingly takes, entices, or keeps from lawful custody any child under 18 years of age who is legally entrusted to the custody of another person or institution. Violation of this law in one state, for example, is a misdemeanor if committed by the noncustodial parent or an agent of the parent and if the child is voluntarily returned unhurt; it is a felony if the child is injured or involuntarily returned. Custodial interference by all other persons under any circumstance also is a felony. Thus, an MHP should ensure that divorce and separation decrees and agreements permit the noncustodial parent to request and be responsible for the treatment before agreeing to provide services to the noncustodial parent's child.

May Others Consent to a Minor's Treatment?

Some states have enacted laws that allow individuals other than the parents or other entities to give consent for the medical treatment of a minor. For example, parents or guardians can always delegate their authority to consent to other persons or entities (e.g., private educational facilities at which a child is enrolled). In addition, one state's law provides that when the custodial parent or guardian cannot be reached in a timely manner and has not given notice to the contrary, certain individuals may give consent to medical care for a minor, as long as the consent is written and includes certain information (e.g., name of child and parents, name and relationship of person giving consent, and nature and dates of treatment). The people who can give consent under this rule include grandparents, adult brothers and sisters, and adult aunts and uncles. Courts may also appoint a guardian *ad litem* with the power to consent in limited areas such as mental health services, even though the parent still maintains parental authority in all other areas (see chap. 6). Finally, at least one state allows peace officers who have lawfully taken custody of a minor and who have reasonable grounds to believe that the minor is in immediate need of medical treatment (e.g., emergency mental health treatment) to consent to the needed services.

FEES, BILLING, AND COLLECTION ARRANGEMENTS

Because the MHP–client relationship is an economic and contractual one and not just therapeutic, MHPs should prepare a formal written agreement to protect the rights and interests of both parties at the outset of services. The client has the right to receive confidential, competent, and appropriate services that are performed according to the professional standards of the MHP's discipline and licensure law. In return, the MHP should receive the client's cooperation with the service (e.g., treatment) plan and payment for services rendered. The written contract, therefore, should be drafted according to local laws and serve the following functions:

- clearly establish the fee structure, policies regarding charges and payment (e.g., charges per session and charges for missed sessions), and the client's commitment to paying the MHP;
- describe the nature and scope of services to be provided (see the previous informed consent discussion);
- explain the general rule of confidentiality and its exceptions (see chap. 3); and
- require the client to consent to the agreement by signing it.

What Is the Law Regarding Fees?

A few states require MHPs to have written fee agreements with their clients. In addition, some professional organizations have created standards regarding fee arrangements, violation of which could lead to malpractice liability (see chap. 4). But perhaps most important, by discussing fees and making written fee agreements with clients in advance of service, the MHP will avoid potential disputes in the future, and get a head start in treatment by modeling clear communication and problem-solving skills. For example, when discussing fees and the expectation to be paid, the MHP should ask the client to discuss any problems he or she might anticipate in payment and ensure that the client understands and agrees to the arrangement. By setting and documenting the fee arrangement, one can determine whether the client's financial situation (including insurance coverage) might affect the length of the therapeutic relationship and one's preference for a particular therapeutic modality.

How Should a Mental Health Professional Set Fees?

In most cases, the law does not speak to the fees that an MHP chooses to charge. That is a personal, professional decision. But one's choice of fees can affect the likelihood that one will be compensated by a third-party payer. For example, insurance companies generally reimburse psychologists at the UCR rate.

The fee charged a patient becomes a legal issue if an MHP tries to fraudulently overcharge a third-party payer. For example, consider the situation in which the MHP agrees to charge a patient $100 per hour for his service and the patient is covered by an insurance plan that reimburses only 80% of the fee, leaving the patient to pay the remaining 20%. If the MHP bills the insurance company $130 per hour for the service, rather than the $100, to save the patient from paying anything, the MHP has committed fraud and will be subject to criminal and civil liability. Or, if the MHP bills only the third-party payer for the 80%, forgiving the patient the 20%, the MHP has arguably defrauded the insurance company. In this latter situation, the insurance company could argue that the true cost of the MHP's services was only 80% of the 100% claimed and that the insurance company should only be requested to pay 80% of that 80% billed.

What Are the Issues Involved in Billing and Collection?

In this section, we discuss billing and reimbursement from clients who pay their own bills, rather than relying on a third-party payer. (We discuss clients who use a third-party payer in the next section.)

An MHP can collect fees either by asking the client to pay after each session or by sending the client a bill after he or she leaves the session. It is preferable to collect fees at the time of service as this is the safer way to get paid. If this is not possible, the MHP should suggest that the client make partial payment. Providing clients with the convenience of using credit cards can help make payment easier and has the additional benefit of shifting the burden of collection from the MHP to the credit card company.

If a client becomes delinquent in payment of bills, one has a number of options that one can use to encourage payment, including letters, discreet phone calls, flexible payment plans, a responsible collection agency, and small claims court. State law may restrict use of certain practices, such as disclosing information about a debt to third parties without legal justification. The method chosen should respect one's professional obligations to the client (and patient if not the client), including protecting client confidentiality and avoiding harming the patient. Further, although the MHP has the legal right to pursue payment for services, the decision to do so should be balanced against the direct and indirect costs that he or she will incur if the former client countersues for malpractice or files a disciplinary complaint with the licensure board or an ethics complaint with the state or national disciplinary association (e.g., the American Psychological Association).

Some states outline the procedures an MHP must take before using a collection agency or court to resolve the problem. If an MHP does not practice in one of these states, his or her first response to serious nonpayment should be to write a letter to the client documenting that he or she has not received a response to repeated attempts to secure payment, that he or she is still willing to talk and work something out with the client, but that after a reasonable period of time (e.g., 20 days) legal action will be sought if payment is not made. Never show feelings or displays of personal hostility to the client.

INSURANCE REIMBURSEMENT FOR SERVICE

It is increasingly common that clients are not the ones who pay directly for mental health services. In this section, we discuss the law regarding how MHPs are reimbursed by third-party payers, specifically insurance agencies.

Health insurance carriers (insurers) generally have considerable discretion in defining the scope and nature of mental health service coverage in their policies. In many states, insurance policies limit reimbursement for particular types of problems and services and to certain classes of health care providers. Some of these policies are arguably discriminatory because they include insurance coverage for physical health needs but not mental health needs and because they only reimburse certain types of MHPs.

The states have responded to this problem in a variety of ways. First, state law may prohibit the denial of reimbursement for mental health services in hospital or medical service plan contracts, health care service plan contracts, and disability and group disability insurance contracts. For instance, many states have laws that require the inclusion of some specified minimum level of mental health coverage in all insurance policies offered in that state. In addition, some states mandate that any health insurance plan provided for state government employees include certain mental health benefits. For example, one state's law mandates yearly and lifetime benefits for "mental illness or functional nervous disorders" provided by physicians or licensed psychologists and sets the deductibles that state employees must pay for services. Typically, however, even when the law mandates coverage for mental health services, the benefits provided will be far more limited than that provided for health care services.

Coverage disparity is no longer the norm, however, for some employer benefit programs as a result of the 1996 federal Mental Health Parity Act (MHPA), which applies to employers with 50 or more employees. It provides that if their group health plans include both medical–surgical benefits and mental health benefits, they will not be allowed to set annual or lifetime dollar limits on mental health benefits that are lower than any such limits for medical benefits. However, MHPA protections do not extend to benefits for substance abuse or chemical dependency.

Second, some insurance companies and policies have sought to exclude certain categories of MHPs from their reimbursement provisions. Psychiatrists may receive reimbursement more easily than other MHPs, and it is not uncommon for certain types of MHPs to be excluded from reimbursement coverage completely. If MHPs other than psychiatrists are allowed coverage, the policy may state that to be reimbursed the MHP must satisfy certain conditions (e.g., have authorization or referral from an MD). In response, most states have enacted a law (known as a freedom of choice law) that mandates insurers to reimburse other specified MHPs (e.g., psychologists) if they are going to reimburse psychiatrists. Such laws do not typically include all of the MHP disciplines, however (e.g., counselors).

3

MAINTAINING AND DISCLOSING INFORMATION

Most clients of mental health services consider having their personal information kept private to be extremely important. In this chapter, we consider the legal issues surrounding the maintenance and disclosure of information obtained during the provision of mental health professionals' (MHPs') services. The key concepts and terms that one will need to understand when reading this chapter include confidentiality, privilege, search, seizure, and subpoena.

- A *confidential* communication refers to written or verbal information conveyed by the client to an MHP in the course of a professional relationship. MHPs have a duty to maintain client confidentiality; however, it is subject to various exceptions.
- *Privileged* communication refers to the right of the client to maintain the confidentiality of information in legal proceedings. Confidentiality law does *not* apply to such proceedings, so states had to enact privileged communications statutes to extend confidentiality into the courtroom.
- A *search* refers to the on-site investigation by a law enforcement officer of a person or a person's property. Although a search

is typically used in the investigation of criminals, MHPs may be searched either because the police believe that the MHP has committed a criminal act (e.g., billing fraud) or because a client of the MHP is being investigated.

- *Seizure* refers to the acquisition of physical information (e.g., written records and case files) that was identified through a search.
- *Subpoena* refers to a document issued by a court, typically at the request of an attorney, for a person (e.g., an MHP) to either appear personally to testify or to provide written records.

EXTENSIVENESS, OWNERSHIP, MAINTENANCE, AND ACCESS TO RECORDS

Records, which are an important part of an MHP's practice, are regulated by the law. States may differ, however, in the way they treat such records. For example, one state's law regulates records kept by psychiatrists and psychologists, but not by other MHPs. Federal law also applies to records of some MHPs (see the section on the Health Insurance Portability and Accountability Act [HIPAA] at the end of this chap.).

How Extensive Do the Records Have to Be?

Maintaining records is not only necessary for the conduct of a good and ethical mental health practice but licensure law generally requires it. For example, state licensure law concerning one's discipline may specify that an MHP engages in unprofessional conduct if he or she fails to maintain adequate business, financial, and professional records on the services that are provided to clients. If there is not a definition of *adequate* in the law, it presumably means sufficient to provide mental health services and to accurately reflect what occurred during services. State law and ethical guidelines may also specify

- the time when the records should be made (e.g., contemporaneous with the service),
- the nature and extent of the professional interaction that should be contained in the record (e.g., location of the service, chief presenting problem of the patient, components of the treatment, and progress evaluations), and
- how additions or corrections to an existing record should be made (e.g., sign and date each change).

Who Owns a Mental Health Professional's Records?

Unless state law specifies otherwise, an MHP may assume that he or she owns his or her records. This does not mean, however, that one may withhold records from one's patient, client, or some other third party. The MHP needs to understand his or her state's confidentiality and privileged communications law to know who has the legal right to access patient records, to what extent, and under what conditions (see the following sections on access).

How Long Should Records Be Maintained?

State law may or may not specify a minimum period of time for which records must be kept. If the law provides that records must be maintained for a minimum period of years (e.g., 7 years), the period usually starts from the date of the last client activity. If the records are relevant to an investigation by the licensure board or a law enforcement agency, the records should be kept until the board or agency provides written notification that the investigation has been completed. This may take longer than the minimum period of years.

State law may also specify the procedures to follow to maintain the confidentiality of client records. These procedures typically ensure that the records are preserved in the case of an MHP's relocation, separation from a group practice, retirement, or death. In addition, the law may also address the use of computers to prepare and maintain client records (e.g., require a write-protected program). Generally, however, one is likely to be considered a prudent provider if one takes reasonable precautions (i.e., precautions that similar MHPs would take) to protect clients' records.

What Access Do Clients Have to Records?

State law may or may not specify what access clients have to the records. Although most states hold that MHPs must make records available to clients on request, laws may vary as to whether the request needs to be in writing, if fees may be charged for the service (e.g., for time spent copying records), and if there are limits on what type of information and in what format one may provide the requested information. For example, depending on the state, the record may be withheld, given in summary form, or have parts removed (e.g., with a black marker) if release of the record would harm the client (e.g., adversely and substantially affect the client's mental health or well-being). State law may hold that psychologists may exclude raw test data and psychometric testing materials when providing records to clients. Last, state law may or may not give minors a right of access to their records.

Will the State Licensure Board Have Access to a Mental Health Professional's Records?

State law usually specifies when an MHP must divulge client information, including records about the client. One such circumstance is when the licensure board investigates an MHP. These boards typically have broad powers to investigate any activities pertaining to the enforcement of the licensure law and one's practice that come under their purview (see chap. 1).

Do Hospital Review Boards Have Access to Records?

Certain hospitals are required to have a utilization review committee to review the professional practices within the hospital for the purposes of reducing morbidity and mortality and for the improvement of patient care. Although this law does not mandate disclosure of records, utilization review committees usually have access to all hospital records concerning the care and treatment of all patients. Thus, records documenting mental health services delivered in a hospital would be available to the review committee, although the law may specify that patient identifiers be removed prior to the review committee's receiving the records.

Will There Be Liability for Violation of Records Law?

Violation of records laws may result in suspension or revocation of one's license or in some other sanction by the licensure board and may result in civil or criminal liability (see chap. 4).

CONFIDENTIAL RELATIONS AND COMMUNICATIONS

Generally, a confidential communication is written or verbal information conveyed by the client to an MHP in the course of a professional relationship. Confidentiality originated in professional ethics codes and arose from a belief that effective psychotherapy required a guarantee from the therapist that no information obtained in the course of patient evaluation or treatment would be given to others without the client's consent. In general, state law has adopted this approach to confidentiality for psychologists and psychiatrists; the law varies from state to state on whether this standard is extended to other MHPs.

Is Confidentiality Absolute?

Confidentiality and the duty to maintain it are not absolute. As already noted, confidential information is not protected in legal proceedings unless a privileged communications law in one's state protects it. In addition, MHPs may not be able to use the duty of confidentiality as an excuse to fail to take actions that may be necessary to protect the patient, client, or others in society. For example, there is an exception to confidentiality for psychologists if the client presents a clear and imminent danger to herself or himself and refuses to accept further treatment. Other confidentiality exceptions discussed in later sections in this chapter include

- protecting third parties from dangerous persons;
- reporting criminal activity;
- confidentiality with HIV-positive patients;
- reporting child abuse;
- reporting adult abuse;
- reporting unprofessional conduct by other practitioners;
- search, seizure, and subpoena; and
- HIPAA.

Information also may be released if the client sues the MHP. It would be unfair to allow a patient to sue an MHP for malpractice (see chap. 4) but not allow the MHP to defend her- or himself in court by introducing the patient's treatment records. Finally, if the client gives his or her written consent to a release of information, typically the MHP must release the records unless it is likely to harm the patient. Thus, it is important that MHPs inform clients of the limits of confidentiality at the initiation of services.

What Is the Liability for Violation?

Several types of penalties may be imposed for violations of confidentiality. First, as previously noted, licensure law provides that the licensure board may suspend or revoke the license of any person betraying professional confidences or it may impose other penalties such as probation (i.e., allowing continued practice subject to certain conditions such as seeing a therapist). The same offending actions may also subject the MHP to criminal penalties or a civil lawsuit by the client (see chap. 4).

CONFIDENTIALITY WHEN THE PATIENT IS A MINOR

As discussed in chapter 2, one needs to know who is the client, and thus, who has the right to consent to services. An MHP's duty to maintain confidentiality is owed to the client, who is not necessarily the patient. In reference to therapy with a minor, this means that, in the typical case, information concerning the mental health services is available to the client (e.g., the parent) and unavailable to anyone else without the client's consent. Thus, the minor could be barred access to his or her own records. The reverse is also true; if the state law allowed the minor to be the client and consent to the services (e.g., because the minor is emancipated under state law), then the parent would not typically get access without the minor's consent. The logic is that one cannot share information (records or verbal information) with third parties without the consent of the client (i.e., the one who legally consented to the services).

Although how the law works is relatively easy to describe, state approaches vary. For example, a state may mandate that parents who are not clients be given information about their child's progress in therapy, and conversely, a state could grant some minors (e.g., those above a certain age) the right to access their records even if they were not the consenting party. Granting a third party access to records without client approval or withholding access to records when the law mandates the right to that access makes one vulnerable to a malpractice suit or civil or criminal liability (see chap. 4).

PRIVILEGED COMMUNICATIONS

Two primary areas of law exist to protect the client's communications from disclosure. As discussed in the previous sections, the most well-known is confidentiality law, whose principles originated in professional ethics codes and have now been incorporated in legislation and court rulings. Although confidentiality law protects the client from improper disclosure of information by the MHP in most situations, it does not protect the client from court orders requiring the MHP to disclose information in legal proceedings. For protection in the courtroom, the communications must be covered under a privileged communications statute.

What Is the Privilege?

All states have privileged communications laws, although they vary by the type of MHP discipline covered and the scope of the privilege. Some states only have laws that pertain to psychologists and psychiatrists, whereas other states have laws that apply to a wider variety of MHP disciplines. If there is no privileged communications law for particular MHP disciplines in some states, their clients' disclosures may be revealed in a court hearing if the MHP is asked to testify.

The scope of the privilege varies; some states have separate privileged communications laws that list the covered communications, whereas others provide the same protections to MHPs as provided in the state's attorney–client or physician–patient (which also covers psychiatrists) privileged communications law. Whatever approach to granting privilege is used, it typically covers communications made by the client (and patient) to the MHP and advice the MHP gave the client (and patient) in the course of their professional relationship. States do vary, however, in what the privilege covers. For example, one state recognizes a privilege for mental health information in civil cases, but not for criminal cases.

If a communication is privileged, the MHP must not divulge the information without the consent of the client. The privilege also covers the MHP's employees who come into contact with confidential information obtained in the scope of their employment.

How Does a Mental Health Professional Assert or Waive the Privilege?

The privilege belongs to the client and not the MHP. Thus, only the client may waive the privilege. This holds true even after termination of services. In the case of the client's death, the client's legal heir may assert the privilege. The court or examining attorney will not raise the question of privilege; however, the MHP has the obligation to raise the issue of privilege. If he or she does not, the court or examining attorney will require the MHP to testify. This is particularly problematic because the MHP will be vulnerable to a malpractice suit by the client for breach of privilege if he or she reveals privileged information.

Once the privilege issue is raised by the MHP, a court must determine whether a privilege exists on the basis of several criteria. First, the court will consider whether the MHP's credentials meet the legal requirements for the operation of the privilege. The credentialing requirement is often determined by whether the MHP complied with the licensure law. Second, the court will not assume that the MHP has seen the client in a professional capacity. Thus, there must be a showing that the client (patient) sought mental health services for diagnosis, evaluation, or treatment and that the communication between the MHP and the client (patient) took place in a professional relationship. Third, the court will consider whether the client has waived the privilege. This is important because the privileged communications statutes were designed solely to protect the client; when that person waives the privilege, the communications are no longer protected. Thus, an MHP cannot refuse to release information to the court once the client has waived the privilege. The client may waive the protections of the privilege either expressly in a written document or implicitly. There is an implied waiver when

- the MHP needs to defend him- or herself against a client's lawsuit alleging malpractice,
- a client consults with an MHP in the presence of a third party who is not the MHP's employee or consultant on the case (unless a state law specifically grants the privilege in this situation), or
- the client voluntarily releases the professional information to a third party (e.g., a friend) who is not legally entitled to that information.

What Are the Exceptions to the Privilege?

States have enacted different statutory exceptions to the privilege. In addition to express and implied waivers of the privilege (as previously described), such exceptions generally include

- judicial or administrative proceedings brought against the MHP by the client;
- judicial or administrative proceedings brought against the MHP by the licensing board;
- criminal trials in which the client defendant raises a mental status defense;
- civil trials in which the client's mental condition is an issue;
- civil commitment proceedings against a client;
- proceedings against the client involving claimed abuse or neglect of minors, adults, or an institutionalized patient;
- child custody disputes in which the client's mental health is in question in regard to fitness for custody; and
- judicial proceedings in which the MHP is appointed by the court to examine a criminal defendant to determine whether the defendant is competent to proceed in the criminal process (see chaps. 12, 13, and 14) or to investigate the defendant's mental condition at the time of the offense (see chap. 13).

What Is the Liability for Violation?

MHPs who improperly testify may face civil liability for violation of the privileged communication. Thus, an MHP should always assert the privilege prior to testifying and then ask the court to provide the MHP with a written order forcing disclosure. The trial court's order requiring the MHP to testify would protect him or her against liability relating to the testimony.

PROTECTING THIRD PARTIES FROM DANGEROUS PEOPLE

As noted previously, MHPs' duty of confidentiality is not absolute. This section discusses MHPs' duties to protect third parties from dangerous patients. Such duties compete with and often limit MHPs' duty of confidentiality. Specifically, MHPs who engage in therapy with patients may have a duty to use reasonable standards and methods to diagnose dangerousness and a duty to protect (or in some states warn) foreseeable victims, intended victims, and those in close relationship to them. Typically this duty arises if the patient has communicated a threat of (imminent) serious physical violence against a readily identifiable individual (including the patient) and if the circumstances are such that a reasonable practitioner would believe that the patient intended to carry out the threat or that the patient intended to commit such an act even without a specific threat. Some states have also extended the duty to protection of property.

The specifics of which MHPs incur this duty and who the MHPs must protect vary by state. For example, some only require protection of a specifically identified intended victim. Others make the duty much broader and extend the duty to protect to reasonably foreseeable victims who would be near the intended victim (e.g., students in a classroom in which the teacher is the intended victim).

Typically, the MHP can discharge this duty to protect by

- arranging for voluntary or involuntary hospitalization of the patient,
- advising local law enforcement of the threat and the identity of the intended victim(s),
- warning the intended victim(s), or
- warning the parent if the intended victim(s) are minors.

If state law requires MHPs to protect a third party from dangerous patients and if MHPs act on that legal obligation, this constitutes a legal exception to confidentiality requirements. A patient cannot sue an MHP for breach of confidentiality for protecting the intended victim if state law required the MHP's action. When a patient's statements are no longer confidential, they will not be privileged. Thus, the MHP would be able to testify in court about the patient's statements made in therapy that led to the warnings or other protective actions.

MHPs need to understand whether their state imposes a duty to assess for potential violence and to protect or warn potential victims from the future actions of their clients. MHPs may face a professional negligence suit if they do not protect or warn third parties as prescribed in their state's law. However, MHPs may face a breach of confidentiality lawsuit (see chap. 4) if they disclose threats of violence to a range of possible victims who are not protected by the law.

REPORTING PAST CRIMINAL ACTIVITY

A few states require MHPs to report to law enforcement officials knowledge of a client's past crimes. Failure to report this information may result in criminal or civil penalties. In such cases, the MHP would not be liable to the client for breach of confidentiality because the report would be considered a legally valid exception to confidentiality.

Most states, however, do not require MHPs to report such information, although psychiatrists, like all other physicians, may be required to report patients' gunshot wounds. If the MHP provides past crime information voluntarily (i.e., without a court order to do so), he or she may be sued by the patient for breach of confidentiality (see chap. 4). In these states, for example, if an MHP is asked by a government official (e.g., a child protective services [CPS] worker or a police officer) to relay information about the past crimes of a patient, the MHP should not do so without ensuring that the information is no longer confidential. If an MHP chooses to respond, he or she should not give false information as this may result in criminal prosecution (e.g., for obstruction of justice).

REPORTING ONGOING OR PLANNED CRIMINAL ACTIVITY

Another exception to MHPs' duty of confidentiality can arise in situations in which criminal activity is ongoing or planned. In general, state legislators do not want to impose law enforcement investigatory obligations on MHPs, and therefore, do not require the reporting of ongoing or planned crimes. Yet three sources of law suggest that the states may be moving in this direction. First, MHPs often incur these obligations under existing specific reporting obligations, such as reporting ongoing child abuse or protecting third parties and their property from dangerous persons. Second, some states allow MHPs to breach confidentiality to prevent the continuation of a serious ongoing crime or the execution of a serious planned crime, and at least one state rules that there is no confidentiality for this information. Thus, if law enforcement hears of the information and wants it, the MHP has no legal ground to withhold it in those states. Third, at least one state requires reporting when an MHP discovers that his or her client is using the MHP's services or is seeking the services of another MHP to aid someone else in the commission of a crime (e.g., seeking mental health services to help establish a fraudulent insanity defense to a criminal act). Finally, the law has not addressed the case in which one's client reveals that although he or she committed a crime, another person was convicted and is serving a sentence for that crime.

CONFIDENTIALITY WITH HIV-POSITIVE PATIENTS

Patients with HIV cannot be confident that their status will be confidential. Every state requires all new HIV-positive test results (not names of these cases) to be reported to a governmental agency. However, some states require this disclosure to include the names of those people with HIV but charge the agency to keep such information confidential. In addition, some states require the name of the patient with HIV to be reported to sexual partners of the person. If the patient is a minor, some states allow him or her to be treated for venereal disease without parental consent, whereas others require or allow parents to be notified and to give consent.

Is There a Duty to Warn Partners of HIV-Positive Patients?

At this time, MHPs in most states have no clear legal duty to warn or to protect sexual partners of their clients who have been diagnosed with HIV/ AIDS or AIDS-related complex (ARC). However, some states have created an exception to the duty of confidentiality in these cases. For example, one state permits disclosure to medical or law enforcement personnel when an MHP determines that the patient with an infectious disease poses a probability of imminent physical harm to others. In addition, health care professionals are required to notify that state's partner protection program when the professional knows the patient is HIV positive and presents a risk of transmission to a third party. The professional also may release results of an HIV test to the spouse of the person tested. Because the law is constantly changing and moving in the direction of limiting confidentiality in this area, MHPs should, as a matter of sound practice,

- check the law in their state to determine whether it has addressed this issue and what the law requires and permits,
- attempt to persuade the patient to take precautions against transmission of the disease,
- advise the patient to let any sexual partners know of the possible risk,
- consider informing uncooperative clients that they may be held liable in a civil or criminal lawsuit for knowingly transmitting a sexual disease to another person, and
- document that they have made such efforts to act as a reasonable and ethical MHP.

What Is the Liability for Violation?

If one's state requires reporting of patients with infectious diseases, including HIV/AIDS or ARC, the MHP may be criminally and civilly liable for violating that law by not reporting. We say *may* because some states by statute provide immunity for MHPs who fail to make the required notification to a relevant state agency.

One can be sued even if state law requires that an MHP divulge patient information to protect a third party (e.g., the partner of the patient with HIV). Angry clients may claim that the MHP breached confidentiality. They will not win the suit, however, because confidentiality did not exist if the MHP's state imposes a reporting obligation. Finally, third parties may claim that the MHP had a duty to warn them (because they were reasonably foreseeable victims) to avoid serious physical and emotional injury (see the discussion in this chap. on the duty to protect third parties).

REPORTING CHILD ABUSE

Although all states allow the use of reasonable discipline that does not harm a child's health, welfare, or safety, they require MHPs to report various kinds of known or suspected abuse of children, including sexual abuse, physical abuse, emotional abuse, and neglect. Abuse may also include children who are born physically dependent on addictive drugs and newborns who have been deprived of life supporting materials. In addition, some states have laws that require the reporting of prior abuse of a child who is now an adult.

Who Must Report Child Abuse?

State laws differ on who is required to report child abuse. Some states impose the duty broadly to include any person who reasonably believes a child is being abused. Other states require only certain professionals, including MHPs, who have professional contact with the child to report known or suspected abuse. Thus, in these latter states, providing services to an alleged abuser of a child would not trigger a duty to report. When the MHP does have a duty to report, most states do not require these MHPs to be licensed; thus, all MHPs may have a legal duty to report child abuse when they otherwise meet the requirements for reporting under the law.

How Does a Mental Health Professional Make a Report of Child Abuse?

The duty to report is usually discharged by a report to the appropriate state agency (e.g., law enforcement or CPS). State law usually requires that a report be made immediately or within a minimum period of time (e.g., 2 days) after the MHP knows of or suspects the abuse. If initial reports are made in person or by telephone, a follow-up written report is often required within a certain time (e.g., 48 hours). The report generally should include the following information:

- the name, address, telephone number, and occupation of the person reporting;
- the name, address, and age of the minor;
- the names and addresses of the minor's parents or other persons with custody of the child;
- the nature and the extent of the injury(ies), abuse, and neglect;
- any evidence of previous occurrences or injuries;
- any statement related to the incident made by the victim;

- the names of any individuals believed to have knowledge of the abuse;
- the names of any individuals believed to be responsible for the abuse and their connection to the victim; and
- any other information the reporting person believes will be helpful in establishing the cause of the abuse.

What Liability Does the Mental Health Professional Encounter in This Area?

Complying with child abuse reporting laws is mandatory. Failure to follow these laws may result in criminal sanctions, and civil liability from the victimized party this law is designed to protect.

Some states provide explicit legal protection for MHPs who comply with a child abuse reporting law. In addition, most child abuse reporting laws include an immunity provision that protects a person from reporting suspected child abuse, even if there was no explicit duty to report. MHPs reporting under such laws will be immune from employment sanctions, criminal liability, and civil liability, unless the MHP acted with malice against the alleged abuser. Malice usually refers to the intent to inflict an injury, though it sometimes includes recklessness. Thus, when an MHP makes a report based on obviously incorrect information, the law may infer malice, even though there is no specific intent to injure a particular person.

REPORTING ADULT ABUSE

Some states require certain professionals, including MHPs, to report known or suspected abuse, neglect, or exploitation of elder, dependent, or incapacitated adults. This type of law was designed to protect elderly or disabled adults from harm, and creates another exception to confidentiality and privilege laws. Although each state's definition differs, abuse and neglect generally refer to behavior resulting in physical or emotional harm, whereas exploitation concerns behavior resulting in economic loss.

Who Must Report Adult Abuse?

State law differs on who is required to report adult abuse. Some states have imposed the duty broadly. For example, one state requires any person to report to the appropriate state agency if he or she has reasonable cause to believe that the elderly or disabled person is being abused, neglected, or exploited. Thus, this state requires all MHPs, licensed or not, to report cases of reasonably suspected abuse. Other states require MHPs to report in narrower circumstances, such as abuse occurring in an institutional setting (e.g., hospitals or nursing homes). Finally, some states require reporting by people who have a special relationship with the protected person. For instance, one state imposes the duty to report on persons with responsibility for incapacitated adults and on certain other professionals (i.e., physicians, psychologists, and social workers).

How Does a Mental Health Professional Make a Report of Adult Abuse?

State law usually requires that a report be made immediately or within a short period of time (e.g., 2 days) after the MHP knows of or suspects the abuse, neglect, or exploitation. If initial reports are made in person or by telephone, a follow-up written report is often required within a certain time (e.g., 48 hours). The recipient of the report will vary among and within states. Most states require reports to go to the local adult protective services agency or law enforcement agency. Exploitation may also be reported to the state's office of the public fiduciary. The report generally should include the following information:

- the name, address, telephone number, and occupation of the person reporting;
- the name and address of the victim;
- the age of the victim and the nature and extent of the incapacity, if applicable;
- the nature and the extent of the abuse, neglect, or exploitation;
- any statement related to the incident made by the victim;
- the names of any individuals believed to have knowledge of the incident(s);
- the names of any individuals believed to be responsible for the incident and their connection to the victim; and
- any other information the reporting person believes will be helpful in establishing the cause of the abuse.

REPORTING UNPROFESSIONAL CONDUCT BY OTHER PRACTITIONERS

In the course of a therapeutic relationship, the MHP may learn from the patient about the unprofessional conduct of another MHP whom the patient went to previously. Consider the case in which a client informs her current MHP of a sexual relationship she had with her previous MHP. In one state, the law requires the therapist to keep the information confidential unless the client authorizes disclosure. The therapist in that state is only legally obligated to (a) provide the patient with a booklet entitled *Sexual*

Intimacy Is Never Okay, which discusses the illegality of such conduct as well as the remedies that the patient may choose to pursue, and (b) discuss with the patient the option of her reporting the conduct to the appropriate state licensure board. In another state, however, the MHP may be required to report the unprofessional conduct to the relevant licensing board.

Ethically, the MHP has to balance the duty to prevent serious unethical and illegal conduct with the duties to treat other professionals with respect and not to violate patient confidentiality. If the patient provides the MHP with consent to report the prior violation or if the law or professional ethics requires one to report, the report should be made to the ethics committee of the offending MHP's professional organization and to the relevant state licensure board.

SUBPOENA, SEARCH, AND SEIZURE

During a civil or criminal case, the court may demand information from an MHP that was obtained during the course of a professional relationship with a client. This demand will usually come through a subpoena requesting that an MHP come to court to testify or submit certain records to the court.

Courts also may issue a search warrant authorizing law enforcement to search an MHP's office for information and to seize relevant evidence. The search of an MHP's office and seizure of any records may occur during a criminal investigation of the MHP or of the MHP's clients. Our discussion in this section is limited to the latter situation because the former situation rarely occurs.

Both subpoenas and searches are important to MHPs because they provide exceptions to confidentiality and privileged communications law. However, just because an MHP's records have been subpoenaed or seized, the records may not necessarily be admissible in court. The judge will make that determination at trial (see the following discussion).

How Do Subpoenas Work?

A subpoena is a written order of the court compelling a witness to appear and give testimony or present written documents (e.g., books, papers, documents, and other tangible things in the possession or control of the witness). In the case of subpoenaed verbal testimony, the court order must contain the name of the court, title of the legal case, and the time and place where the testimony is to be given. In the case of subpoenaed written documentation, the court order must specify the documentation sought and to where and when it is to be delivered.

A subpoena is put into effect (served) when a copy is delivered directly to the witness and when fees for 1 day's attendance and mileage allowed by law have been offered. (Some states allow criminal defendants or the indigent the right to compel testimony without paying witness or mileage fees.) Failure to appear at the time and place specified in the subpoena may result in contempt of court proceedings, which can lead to the MHP being jailed until the MHP consents to appear in court. Note that if one is not subpoenaed but chooses for some other reason to attend a court hearing, this can result in the MHP being requested to testify in the same manner as if subpoenaed!

An MHP may be compelled to testify at a court hearing or deposition or by a public officer or entity authorized to take evidence (e.g., a licensure board). But if an MHP as a witness finds that the subpoena commands production of documentary evidence that would be unreasonable and oppressive to provide, he or she may make a motion to quash or modify the subpoena. In a civil suit, an MHP as a witness may make a motion to condition compliance upon payment of the reasonable cost of producing the evidence.

The mere issuance of a subpoena does not mean that the privilege is automatically nullified. Rather, the MHP must assert the privilege, unless the client expressly waives it. Once the MHP asserts the privilege, the court will do one of several things: (a) order disclosure of the information and nullify the privilege in this situation, (b) waive the privilege as a matter of law (e.g., because the client disclosed the information in such a way as to extinguish its confidential nature), or (c) agree with the MHP that the privilege overcomes the subpoena and modify or quash the subpoena. Failure by an MHP to assert the privilege initially may result in civil or criminal liability for breach of confidence if it is likely that the court would have upheld the privilege and quashed the subpoena.

How Does Search and Seizure Work?

Search and seizure law refers to a governmental official's search or seizure of things or places. Search and seizure is typically authorized by a written order (i.e., a search warrant) from a judge or magistrate (i.e., a lower judicial official) directing the governmental officer to search for specific items. Although warrantless searches are sometimes permissible, such searches are generally restricted to extreme circumstances. Thus, it is unlikely that an MHP would be subjected to a warrantless search.

A request for a search warrant will be granted when the judge is satisfied that there is probable cause that the objects of the search exist at the specified location. The applicant must give the judge facts via an affidavit or sworn testimony, and the facts must support the grounds for application of the search warrant, which names the relevant persons and describes the relevant items and places with specificity. The warrant identifies the property to be seized, describes the person or place to be searched, and specifies the hours when it may be executed. In addition, it may specify the reasons for issuing the search warrant. For example, one state's law provides that a search warrant may be issued when the property (e.g., documents, papers, and books) to be seized

- was stolen or embezzled,
- was used as a means of committing a public offense,
- is in the possession of a person having the intent to use it as a means of committing a public offense or of another person to whom she or he may have delivered it for the purpose of concealing it or preventing it from being discovered, or
- consists of any item that tends to show that a particular public offense has been committed or that a particular person has committed the public offense.

It is this last reason that is typically used to search and seize the MHP's records concerning a particular client.

Generally, the search warrant must be executed (used) within a certain period of time (e.g., 5 days in one state, 10 in another) after its issuance. State law also may differ as to how the warrant may be executed. One state provides that the officer may break into the building if either no response is received within a reasonable time or, after notice of their authority and purpose, the officers are refused admittance. Another state allows the officer to enter without an announcement to execute the warrant if the officer has reason to believe that an announcement would result in the destruction of the property. Further, some states allow officers to search any person if it appears that the sought property is concealed on the person.

Some states require the officer to give a copy of the warrant and a receipt for the seized property to the person from whom the property is taken or leave a copy of the warrant if no one is present. Other states do not require the officer to serve a copy of the warrant before or at the time of the search. Instead, such states require the officer only to issue a detailed receipt of any property taken. Persons objecting to any aspect of a search should contact their attorney because police officers may respond with appropriate force to execute the search warrant. If there remains a dispute regarding seized property, the MHP may request a court hearing to determine the legality of the search or seizure (e.g., if there was probable cause to seize the item and if the property was the same as described in the search warrant). If the search was illegal, the property would be restored to the MHP and would not be permitted as evidence in court. However, this will not always protect the information from being seen by law enforcement officials, which may pose a problem for certain high-profile patients (e.g., celebrities and public officials).

PEER REVIEW ACTIVITIES

In addition to regulating the work of hospital review committees (discussed earlier), the law regulates the ability of third-party payers (insurance companies) to obtain treatment information about MHP's patients. The insurance companies use this information to determine the appropriateness of paying the MHP and the amount of payment. If the third-party payer believes that the MHP's treatment is not usual, customary, or reasonable, the payer may request and pay for an independent review by a professional review committee (PRC). The request is generally put in writing to the treating MHP, and the PRC will conduct a confidential review of the case. Typically, the PRC is composed of professionals who match the discipline of the MHP who requested payment. Before the review may begin, clients are usually required to sign a detailed authorization to disclose information to the reviewers.

Typically, peer review law limits the scope of information that may be disclosed to third-party payers. For example, disclosures to third-party payers in one state are limited to

- administrative information;
- diagnostic information;
- status of the patient (e.g., voluntary or involuntary and inpatient or outpatient); and
- rationale for continuing mental health services, which may require an assessment of the patient's current level of functioning and level of distress (e.g. mild, moderate, severe, or extreme).

Third-party payers are typically prohibited from further disclosure of treatment information except when required by law or in legal disputes to settle payment claims.

HEALTH INSURANCE PORTABILITY AND ACCOUNTABILITY ACT

In 2003, federal law effectively established national privacy standards governing the use and disclosure of "protected health information" that includes most mental health information by "covered entities." Covered entities are health plans, health care clearinghouses, and any health care provider who transmits health information in electronic form in connection with transactions for which the U.S. Secretary of Health and Human Services has adopted standards under HIPAA (e.g., claims, benefit eligibility inquiries, and referral authorization requests). For help in determining who or what is a covered entity, consult the decision tool at http://www.cms.hhs.gov/hipaa/hipaa2/support/tools/decisionsupport/default.asp. The law is contained in the privacy rule of HIPAA. HIPAA establishes minimum standards regarding the use and disclosure of confidential information as well as the creation of patient rights governing access to records. It also establishes notice provisions that help to ensure that patients are informed about their rights under this law.

HIPAA generally takes the place of state law (i.e., preempts) unless the state law is "more stringent" than the federal law. A state law is more stringent than HIPAA if it provides greater privacy protection for the patient through limitations on disclosure or more powerful patient rights over control of and access to the patient's information. In most states the differences between HIPAA requirements and the existing state law governing confidential information is relatively small. As a rule of thumb, practices consistent with state law will meet or exceed HIPAA requirements if those practices limit the disclosure of all information unless authorized by the patient in writing (except in cases involving abuse, bodily danger to others, or court orders) and provide patient access to the records (except when such access creates a clear danger).

MHPs are generally required to provide access to patients for their records. In addition, under HIPAA, patients have the right to

- restrict disclosure of records to others,
- request amendments to correct inaccurate records,
- receive an accounting of disclosures made over a 6-year period, and
- file a complaint about inappropriate disclosure or use of their records.

A person with legal authority to act on behalf of the patient may exercise these rights. Further, the rights survive the death of the patient.

HIPAA requires covered MHPs to develop and implement written privacy policies and procedures and then train personnel (e.g., office staff and interns) on them. HIPAA also requires MHPs to provide patients with a "privacy notice" that describes the typical uses and disclosures of information for treatment and payment, disclosures that may be made without patient authorization, and a statement that all other disclosures require the patient's revocable written authorization. MHPs generally must obtain written acknowledgment that the patient received the privacy notice.

Under HIPAA, valid authorizations to release information must include

- identification of the person or entity to receive the information,
- who is authorized to disclose,
- the purpose for disclosure,
- the information to be disclosed,
- an expiration date or event,
- a statement that the authorization may be revoked, and
- a dated signature.

MHPs may disclose confidential information without a HIPAA authorization in a variety of circumstances that may be characterized either as an implied consent by the patient or needed to facilitate governmental functions. For example, implied consent is typically assumed when the patient sues the MHP or brings a complaint against the MHP (e.g., for malpractice). If there is any serious question about whether there is a valid implied consent in a particular circumstance, one should apply to a proper court for a court order for the release of the information. This order will protect one from liability. The latter category, facilitating governmental functions, includes complying with mandatory reporting laws (e.g., child abuse reporting), licensing board inquiries, and public health requests and averting a serious threat to public safety.

"Psychotherapy notes," also called process notes, are defined under HIPAA as

> notes recorded (in any medium) by a health care provider who is a mental health professional documenting or analyzing the contents of conversation during a private counseling session or a group, joint, or family counseling session and that are separated from the rest of the individual's medical record.

Although other information may be released to insurers after the patient signs the privacy notice, psychotherapy notes generally require additional written authorization to be released.

4

LIABILITIES FOR
PROFESSIONAL ACTIVITIES

Mental health professionals (MHPs) as individuals or as members of organizations (i.e., licensure boards and ethics committees) are liable for their professional activities. Complaints may be filed against them through their professional organizations or through civil and criminal lawsuits. In this chapter, we discuss the different types of professional, civil, and criminal liability that MHPs may face for problems with their clients, patients, and third parties.

MALPRACTICE LIABILITY

Violations of the licensure law or other failures to act competently may result in civil lawsuits against the MHP. The most common of these legal claims is for malpractice. The client (the plaintiff) in a malpractice suit alleges that he or she suffered a physical, mental, or financial injury because an MHP did not exercise the level of ordinary and reasonable care practiced by the average member of that discipline in the same or similar community. Professional practices that can be legally challenged include all actions of the MHP that directly involve the client and patient and are part of the professional relationship or part of the MHP's professional obligation to the client and patient. For example, in one state, the malpractice action may allege negligence (whether by error or omission), misconduct (which concerns intentional misbehavior), breach of contract (failure to meet the obligations of a written contract to provide services), or failure to obtain express or implied consent before rendering services (see chap. 2). The MHP may also be sued, under the doctrine of *respondeat superior*, for an assistant's or trainee's negligence if the MHP exercises direction and control (i.e., supervises) the assistant or trainee (see chap. 1).

Where Is the Malpractice Suit Tried?

A malpractice claim will be filed by the plaintiff (e.g., the MHP's ex-patient) in the court of general jurisdiction (e.g., the superior court or circuit court) of a state. In some states, whenever a complaint alleges malpractice, the matter must first be considered by a medical liability review panel unless all parties agree to pursue the matter directly in court or if the total damage is less than a certain dollar amount (e.g., $50,000). The panel may appoint a neutral MHP to discuss the pros and cons of the case with the ex-client (plaintiff) and his or her attorney and then conduct an informal hearing to determine if the evidence supports the plaintiff or the defendant. Then, the parties may either settle or proceed with the litigation back in the lower court. Although the panel's decision may be entered into evidence, the finding is not binding on the court's decision. As an alternative to using a liability review panel, some states require the plaintiff to file an affidavit with the court that is accompanied by a written statement from a neutral MHP that the case has merit and should be tried.

Who May Be Sued?

State law provides for who may be subject to a malpractice action. Some states have medical malpractice laws that apply to health care professionals, including MHPs. For example, one state's law defines a licensed health care provider as

> A person, corporation, or institution licensed or certified by the state to provide health care, medical services, nursing services, or other health-related services and includes the officers, employees, and agents thereof working under the supervision of such person, corporation, or institution in providing such health care, medical services, nursing services, and other health-related services.

This means that the individual MHP as well as his or her professional corporation may be the subject of a malpractice suit. In addition, as already noted, any person working under (i.e., supervised by) a certified or licensed MHP who provides health care services comes under this definition, thereby including uncertified psychologists and other related MHPs (see chap. 1) who do not practice independently.

What Is Involved in a Malpractice Suit?

The statute of limitations is the period of time in which a client must file the lawsuit after the alleged malpractice occurred. State laws vary, but generally malpractice suits must be filed within 2 years of the date of the injury or within 2 years of the time that the person knew or should have known facts that would alert the person to the fact that malpractice occurred. The statute of limitations may be extended when the plaintiff is a minor, of unsound mind or incompetent, or imprisoned. In such cases, the law may not start the time period (e.g., 2 years) until the person reaches majority, becomes sane or competent, or is released from prison.

Generally, what needs to be proved in a malpractice suit is determined by a two-part test. First, it must be proved that the MHP failed to exercise that degree of care, skill, and learning expected of a reasonable, prudent health care provider in the discipline (or class of providers to which he or she belongs) acting in the same or similar circumstances. Second, it must be proved that such failure was a cause of the injury (i.e., physical, mental, or financial).

The first element of this test, which refers to the standard of care, means that each MHP will be compared with *reasonable* practitioners of the same discipline. Thus, a psychologist in Oklahoma will be held to the standard of care practiced by other like psychologists practicing within that state. However, if the person is a specialist, the standard of care will typically be considered higher. For instance, an MHP working extensively with people with addiction disorders will be held to a standard of care similar to other MHPs in that state and discipline specializing in addictions. What nonspecialists might do will not be considered the appropriate standard of comparison. Note that the standard of care may be different for persons working in rural areas because of their lack of access to certain resources. Finally, many courts are increasingly holding MHPs to a national standard, rather than focusing on a local standard of care.

If more than one MHP is treating the same person, each provider is not liable for the malpractice of the others unless he or she observed the wrongful act or omission or should have been aware of it in the exercise of ordinary care. Thus, a psychiatrist has the right to rely on the test results, opinions, or other information from an independent psychologist without being responsible for the psychologist's malpractice in the testing.

Evidence of malpractice must be established by expert testimony unless it is so grossly apparent that a layperson would have no difficulty in recognizing it. Usually, this means that the plaintiff must provide testimony by an expert witness in the same discipline stating that the defendant's (i.e., MHP's) actions were below that of the standard of care practiced in the same or similar community. Rather than stating that he or she would have done things differently, the plaintiff's expert witness needs to testify that the method of treatment used by the defendant deviated from the standard of care that would be provided by like professionals.

The next element in the malpractice suit is proof that the defendant's behavior caused the plaintiff's injury. The plaintiff has the burden or responsibility to introduce evidence that affords a reasonable basis for the conclusion that it is more likely than not that the conduct of the defendant was a cause of the plaintiff's injury.

How Can a Mental Health Professional Avoid Malpractice?

So what should an MHP do to avoid malpractice claims and to avoid being hurt by them? There are a number of basic things. An MHP should

- know the rules and regulations promulgated by the licensure board; these rules and regulations constitute a standard of care within that state because all members of the mental health profession are required to follow them (see chap. 1);
- know the standards of care provided by his or her national professional association; these standards are an excellent source of guidance because they typically represent the minimum standard of care;
- know the literature on the particular form of treatment he or she plans to use; the plaintiff's experts are likely to use this literature to challenge the MHP's practice, particularly if he or she plans to use a relatively new, controversial, or unusual technique;
- consult with colleagues and experts; if other colleagues agree in advance, in writing, with the MHP's planned approach, it becomes extremely difficult for the plaintiff to argue that the MHP deviated from what like practitioners would do in this type of case;
- know the results of malpractice lawsuits brought in his or her state; they will inform the MHP about what courts will not tolerate from practitioners;
- carry liability insurance and know the coverage limits of the policy; these policies often limit coverage to acts of negligence and may exclude reimbursement for intentionally wrongful acts or crimes, such as those involving sexual misconduct; and
- consult with his or her malpractice insurer the moment a reasonable fear arises that he or she will be sued.

LIABILITY FOR NONCONSENSUAL TREATMENT

Certain MHP services are so problematic that they can easily generate a liability claim. These situations include forcing services on a client, using aversive conditioning without carefully following one's state's legal regulations regarding the use of these techniques, using invasive treatments, and using research treatment protocols. MHPs who fail to follow the law carefully on these topics may find themselves being subject to penalties imposed by licensure boards and the courts.

Patient's Right to Refuse Treatment

An individual who has the capacity to seek treatment has the capacity to refuse such treatment. In other words, a right to refuse treatment is recognized for people who voluntarily obtain treatment from an MHP.

A right to refuse treatment is not uniformly recognized, however, for persons who have been involuntary committed for services (see chap. 10). And even when the right exists for persons who have been involuntary committed, it will not limit the imposition of services in emergency situations.

May Parents Refuse Treatment for Their Children?

Some states have laws that protect children's right to treatment for life-threatening illnesses. Although these laws were developed to respond to physical medical problems, they could logically be extended to certain life-threatening mental disorders such as pica and severe depression. Where these laws exist, parents of young children cannot refuse treatment for their children, even if the refusal is based on religious objections. The state's interest in protecting children will prevail over the rights of the parents when a determination has been made that the treatment is in the child's best interest.

Regulation of Aversive Conditioning

Despite their demonstrated usefulness in treating people with certain disorders, behavioral therapies using aversive stimuli raise special liability concerns. These therapies include electrical convulsive therapy (ECT) and avoidance conditioning. Avoidance conditioning involves targeting an undesirable response for reduction or elimination and following that response systematically with the presentation of an intense aversive stimulus that results in acute physical discomfort or pain. Some examples of these kinds of aversive stimuli are low-level electric shocks to the patient's arms or legs, physical restraints, the performance of an effortful task, the spraying of a noxious liquid (e.g., lemon juice) in the patient's face, and confinement in a locked room or other isolated area.

States may restrict the nature, scope, and circumstance of aversive conditioning services. For example, one state's law permits such procedures to be used only if two of the three following criteria have been met:

1. The patient exhibits overt self-injurious behavior or is a danger to others.
2. The patient's behavioral problems are so severe or their duration so extensive that other therapeutic approaches are currently precluded or ineffective.
3. Behavior therapy techniques that do not use aversive procedures have been attempted and have failed to remove the problem behavior or behaviors.

Other states require that

- the therapy be approved by an independent MHP, the facility's behavior therapy committee, the facility's manager, or a court;
- the course of treatment be fully described in the patient's individual treatment plan;
- there be on-site state evaluations of facilities using these programs; and
- there be staff training programs for employees who administer these techniques.

Some states have such regulations, but they are only applied to facilities that treat certain populations (e.g., people with developmental disabilities). For example, in one state, the law requires the controlling state agency or department to promulgate rules and regulations concerning the administration of behavioral therapies to persons with developmental disabilities who are served within a state-run or state-supported program. The law of that state also provides for the formation of a human rights committee to provide independent oversight and review to ensure that the rights of the recipients are protected.

For those states without specific laws relating to aversive or avoidance conditioning, MHPs may be held liable for violating a standard of care in conducting such treatments for certain patients in some settings (see the section titled Malpractice Liability at the beginning of this chap.). The more intrusive the treatment, the greater the potential for the MHP to be exposed to liability. The ultimate question in these cases is whether the treatment is generally accepted by like professionals treating similar patients in similar settings.

Regulation of Invasive Treatment Procedures

Some states specifically regulate the use of invasive treatment procedures, including psychosurgery, lobotomy, other brain surgeries, sterilization, and forcibly administered antipsychotic medication, particularly in involuntary cases. Typically, in these cases, such treatment is only allowed if there is a specific informed consent of the patient or legal guardian or an order from the superior court in the county where the treatment is proposed approving with specificity the use of such treatment. A state may also impose specific requirements on invasive procedures. For instance, the state may require that the treatment help the person to function independently and be provided in ways that are the least restrictive of personal liberty.

Regulation of Research as Treatment

When MHPs provide mental health services as part of a research program, ethical and legal regulations may determine the procedures the MHPs must follow. For example, MHPs should obtain informed consent from the potential patients or participants (see chap. 2) that includes potential patients' understanding that they have the right to decline to participate in the study or to withdraw from it at any time. If the MHP researcher is a covered entity, information about the Health Insurance Portability and Accountability Act (HIPAA) must be a part of the informed consent process.

An institutional review board (IRB) also must review and approve such informed consent procedures before the start of any federally funded research project that involves human subjects. The IRB is particularly concerned with protecting vulnerable populations, including children, prisoners, and other institutionalized individuals. When working with young people, MHPs should not only obtain the permission of children's parents or legal guardians but also solicit the agreement (assent) of each child where possible.

In addition to obtaining informed consent from patient participants, MHPs need to protect the confidentiality of the patient participants (see chap. 3). MHPs need to protect these persons' confidentiality because ethical guidelines and law deem any information obtained about a research participant during the course of an investigation to be confidential unless confidentiality was waived. Confidentiality in research becomes a major issue when it comes to publication of the research findings. MHPs should only submit results for publication when patients' identities are completely masked and when patients are made aware of the procedures the MHPs took to safeguard their privacy. MHPs should also consider whether it is in the interest of each patient to have information published about him or her because some individuals may be clinically harmed or may fail to understand what has been written or discussed about their case. Finally, MHPs should be aware of other patient interests. For example, when ongoing data analysis reveals the significant effect of the treatment intervention, the MHP should consider immediately suspending the study to allow the members of the control group to avail themselves of the treatment protocol. MHPs also should avoid continuing to treat a patient just because he or she presents with interesting symptoms.

LIABILITY FOR BREACHING A DUTY TO A THIRD PARTY

As discussed in chapter 3, the law may impose on MHPs certain duties to individuals who are not their clients. Although states may differ, these exceptions to the duty of confidentiality generally include

- protecting third parties from dangerous persons;
- reporting criminal activity;
- confidentiality with HIV-positive patients;
- reporting child abuse;
- reporting adult abuse;
- reporting unprofessional conduct by other practitioners;
- search, seizure, and subpoena; and
- HIPAA.

Third parties may bring a civil suit for malpractice for violating these duties. For example, third parties may claim that an MHP had a duty to warn or otherwise protect them (e.g., because they were reasonably foreseeable victims) from serious physical injury at the hands of his or her patient. As noted earlier (see chap. 3), in cases in which state law requires such a response, doing so is not a breach of confidentiality, and one cannot be sued for divulging what otherwise would be confidential information. MHPs who go beyond the requirements of the law (e.g., disclose threats of violence to a range of possible victims not protected by the law), however, may face a civil lawsuit from their client for breach of confidentiality.

The MHP also may face a criminal lawsuit for breaching a duty to a third party. For example, complying with child abuse reporting laws is mandatory and carries criminal sanctions for noncompliance. Sanctions may also be applied by the licensure board (see chap. 1).

OTHER FORMS OF CIVIL LIABILITY

If a client waits too long to sue on a malpractice theory and is precluded from doing so by the statute of limitations, the claim might be allowed under another legal theory. In addition, lawyers often present alternate legal theories to the judge when bringing the lawsuit to provide the judge or jury choices on which to find in favor of the client and against the MHP. Consider the example of an MHP who wrote a book about a client without the client's permission. The jury did not believe that the MHP committed malpractice because she gave good professional service to the client; but the jury did believe that it was wrong to write a book about the client. If invasion of privacy had been presented as an alternative cause of action to the malpractice claim, the jury could have ruled in favor of the client.

Some types of civil liability are based on MHPs' breaching express or implied responsibilities arising out of the professional relationship (i.e., breach of fiduciary duty and breach of contract). Other types of civil liability are based on intentional actions by the MHP that violate the legal rights of the client (i.e., abandonment; criminal-related actions, such as assault and battery; defamation of character; invasion of privacy; false imprisonment; and abuse of process). Intent is defined as the desire to bring about physical results that the defendant knew or should have known were likely to occur, even if the intent was not hostile. A final type of civil liability is based on intentional actions by the MHP that violate the legal rights of a third party (e.g., defrauding the third-party-payer insurance company or the government). Such an action may also be the basis for a criminal action by the government against the MHP.

What Is Breach of Fiduciary Duty?

The law imposes a fiduciary duty on relationships in which one party is in a superior position to and enjoys the intimate trust of another, with the understanding that the former will act primarily for the latter's benefit. The MHP–client relationship is very likely to be held a fiduciary relationship, although the law in some states may not have addressed this issue yet. If a lawsuit for breach of fiduciary duty is brought, any transactions between the MHP and the client would be very closely examined to determine whether the MHP took advantage of the client. For example, even though a stranger could legally drive a hard bargain with a client over the sale of an item, a court might void an unreasonable service agreement between the MHP and a client who had become dependent on the MHP.

What Is Breach of Contract?

If an MHP contracts to provide services, the MHP will be held liable for failure to live up to that contract. Some states require that the contract be in writing before the client may sue for breach of contract. Thus, in a state with such a law, verbal agreements regarding health care services are unenforceable. MHPs may also be held liable for the breach of a contract with a nonclient (e.g., for failure to pay rent for office space to the landlord).

What Is Abandonment?

Once the MHP–client relationship has been contractually established, the law of abandonment limits the circumstances under which the relationship may be terminated. Generally, the MHP must provide the client with sufficient notice of his or her intent to terminate services to permit the client to obtain the services of another MHP. To facilitate the process and avoid a gap in services, the MHP may be required to assist the client in identifying other MHPs. The MHP may never terminate the client relationship in such a way as to leave the client without the necessary health care in an emergency situation. This situation may require that the MHP participate in contacting another provider on the client's behalf to discharge his or her legal duty to the client.

What Is a Criminal-Related Civil Action?

An MHP who is liable under criminal law (see the next section) may also be liable for the same behavior under civil law. For example, an MHP who is liable for assault and battery under the criminal law may also be liable to the victim for the same behavior under civil law. We say *may* because a jury or a judge in the civil suit may rule differently than the jury or the judge in the criminal case. Thus, the MHP may lose the criminal case but win the civil suit, win the criminal case but lose the civil suit, or win or lose both cases. The difference between a criminal and civil action is that (a) the state prosecutes the MHP in a criminal case, whereas the victim is the plaintiff in a civil case, and (b) the standard of proof in a criminal case is beyond a reasonable doubt, whereas in a civil case it is preponderance of the evidence, which is an easier standard to meet.

If the defendant is found guilty in a criminal case, a penalty of imprisonment or fine is imposed. If the defendant is found liable in a civil action (in a separate trial based on the same facts), a judgment for money damages is rendered. The money is awarded directly to the victim to compensate for actual expenses, such as doctors' bills, lost income, future losses, and for general pain and suffering.

Finally, the criminal courts of some states may order that the MHP pay restitution to the victim only up to the maximum amount of the criminal fine allowed for that offense in that state. Therefore, if the victim had damages that exceeded that amount, the victim would have to sue the MHP in civil court to recover the excess.

What Is Defamation of Character?

Defamation may be either oral (referred to as slander) or written (referred to as libel). In either form, this civil action generally requires that the defendant (i.e., the MHP) communicated information (or caused information to be communicated) about the plaintiff to a third party that caused harm to the plaintiff's reputation and good name. There are two defenses to a defamation suit: (a) the communication was true or (b) the defendant was legally entitled to communicate the information.

What Is Invasion of Privacy?

An invasion of privacy action involves public communication of private information. It requires proof of a public disclosure of private facts that are not matters of public record or generally known and that would be offensive to a reasonable person of ordinary sensibilities. The publication of a book about a client, for example, might give rise to a claim based on invasion of privacy. Note, however, that if an MHP was liable for invasion of privacy, that person usually would, most likely, also have violated ethical principles and laws concerning maintenance of confidences (see chap. 3), and therefore, be subject to a malpractice claim as well.

What Are False Imprisonment and Abuse of Process?

A false imprisonment charge may be brought if a person was physically detained without an authorizing legal order. Some states have a law against excessive detention. The law of one state, for example, allows a client to recover monetary damages against an MHP who knowingly, willfully, or through gross negligence (i.e., wanton or reckless disregard for the rights of others) detained a client in a psychiatric hospital for more than the number of days allowed in the statute. In an abuse of process case, the client alleges that in the course of a legal, justified proceeding, the MHP engaged in some act not authorized by the process or that the MHP engaged in the process because he sought some ulterior objective. An MHP who participated in detaining a person for involuntary commitment without legal justification for doing so or who brought commitment proceedings for reasons not provided for in the state statute would be subject to a false imprisonment charge for the first action and an abuse of process charge for both actions.

The law in some states, however, provides a defense to these actions. For example, the law of one state provides that "any person acting in good faith upon either actual knowledge or reliable information who makes application for evaluation or treatment of another person pursuant to this chapter is not subject to civil or criminal liability for such act." But even without such a statute, MHPs will win these lawsuits if they acted in accordance with accepted professional standards.

What Is Insurance Fraud?

Because some health insurers consider some billing practices by MHPs as fraudulent, they are filing civil lawsuits to recover payments. The law in some states makes it a crime to present a health care payer with a claim for financial reimbursement for services knowing that the claim is fraudulent. Such deceptive practices include lowering the fee for the client but not the insurer and raising the usual and customary fee for billing purposes and then accepting the insurance payment as full payment (see chap. 2).

CRIMINAL LIABILITY

Some states have criminal laws that prohibit MHPs from engaging in certain behaviors (e.g., sexual relations with a client) or that punish MHPs for breaching a legal duty (e.g., failing to report child or elder abuse). Even if state law does not specifically address such issues, there are three general criminal laws (i.e., sex offending, assault and battery, and negligent homicide) that could be of relevance to MHPs because they criminalize behaviors that may arise out of the MHP–client relationship.

What Is the Criminal Law Regarding Sexual Offenses?

State law defines crimes involving sexual offenses. In general, a person commits one of several sexual offenses by engaging in sexual contact or intercourse (any sort of penetration by the penis of the mouth, vulva, or anus or manual masturbatory contact with the penis or vulva) with another individual without his or her consent. *Without consent* generally means that the victim was incapable of consenting because of a variety of factors that may include

- a mental disorder or defect;
- the use of drugs or alcohol, including those administered to the victim without his or her knowledge, that impairs the ability to control or appraise conduct (e.g., so-called *date-rape* drugs);
- being asleep or unconsciousness;
- the physical incapability of resisting;
- coercion with force or threatened use of force against the victim or against another person or property that the victim cares about; and
- the intentional deception of the victim by the offender as to the nature of the act (e.g., deceiving the victim into erroneously believing that the offender was the victim's spouse).

Thus, an MHP who had sexual contact or intercourse with a mentally disordered person could be found guilty of rape. Similarly, masking sexual activity as a treatment or exploiting a client's emotional dependence on the MHP to cause clients to submit to or participate in sexual acts could also be held to be criminal offenses.

What Is the Criminal Law Regarding Assault and Battery?

A person commits assault by intentionally placing another person in reasonable apprehension of imminent physical injury (e.g., threatening them) and battery by intentionally, knowingly, or recklessly causing any physical injury to another person or knowingly touching another person with the intent to injure, insult, or provoke the person. An MHP needs to be concerned about this law because an assault and battery is likely to occur when a therapist touches a client without first obtaining consent. When an owner or employee of a medical or psychiatric institution commits such an offense against one of the residents, the perceived severity of the offense may be increased in the eyes of the judge and jury.

The criminal law, however, permits the use of reasonable force that results in physical injury to another in certain limited circumstances, including

- self-defense—a therapist may use reasonable force to avoid imminent harm to him- or herself;
- defense of another—a therapist may protect a third party in circumstances in which the third party would be justified in using force to protect him- or herself; and
- protection of the client—a therapist may act under a reasonable belief that a client is about to commit suicide or inflict serious injury on him- or herself or others. In these situations, the therapist may use physical force on that person to the extent reasonably necessary to thwart the result.

What Is the Criminal Law Regarding Negligent Homicide?

A person commits negligent homicide if he or she causes the death of someone as a result of criminal negligence. Criminal negligence means that the person failed to perceive a substantial and unjustifiable risk that the result would occur. The risk must be of such nature and degree that failure to perceive it constitutes a gross deviation from what a reasonable person would perceive in the situation. Although the risk usually involves a tangible matter (e.g., when an MHP drives a car well above the speed limit while carrying the client), it presumably could also apply to an MHP who caused a client to become homicidal.

COMPLAINTS BEFORE STATE LICENSURE BOARDS AND NATIONAL AND STATE PROFESSIONAL ETHICS COMMITTEES

As described in chapter 1, when an MHP's client brings a complaint to the attention of the licensure board, that board has broad powers under the law to

- investigate and adjudicate violations of the law,
- specify reasons for sanctioning those found in violation of the law, and
- provide penalties for professionals found in violation.

The penalties chosen by the board may include issuing an educational warning or imposing a sanction on the MHP.

National and state MHP organizations (e.g., the American Psychological Association) have ethics committees that also have the authority to investigate and resolve complaints made about MHPs who are members of that organization. Although there are differences between organizations in the procedures followed, typically they entail the following.

Complaints may be brought before these ethics committees by both members and nonmembers of the professional organization. These complaints are usually required to be in writing, specifying the reason or reasons for bringing the complaint to the committee and authorizing disclosure of material to support the complaint. Alternatively, an ethics committee may be able to investigate on its own initiative when it becomes aware of a potentially serious ethical violation.

Once a complaint has occurred, the committee will carry out a preliminary review to determine whether that discipline's ethics code may have been violated. If it finds in the negative, the committee will dismiss the complaint. If it finds in the affirmative, the committee will advise the accused MHP and ask him or her to reply to the complaint within a certain period of time. The procedures of the ethics committee (e.g., whether the MHP has the right to be represented by counsel, to present witnesses and documents, and to cross-examine witnesses) will be contained in a written policy that is sent to the MHP after the complaint has been filed and an investigation ensues. If after a review of all of the information presented, the ethics committee believes the complaint to be valid and an ethical violation to have occurred, it may

- issue a cease and desist order to the MHP;
- reprimand the MHP;
- censure the MHP;
- require the MHP to have supervision, therapy, or further education;
- impose a probationary period; or
- expel the MHP from membership in the organization.

If the MHP does not accept the decision of the ethics committee, the MHP may appeal the decision to an appeals panel of the organization.

LIABILITY OF CREDENTIALING BOARDS
AND ETHICS COMMITTEES

Certain branches of government, such as the legislature and judiciary, are immune from lawsuits. This originated from the maxim that "the King can do no wrong" but is now premised on the theory that governmental errors that occur during normal governmental activities are better addressed through the ballot box than in the courtroom.

Licensure boards enjoy this sovereign immunity from lawsuit, with limited exception (e.g., violation of federal antidiscrimination laws). Even when such lawsuits are allowed, states in most situations (e.g., if the board members do not act recklessly or grossly negligently) protect board members from having to pay for attorneys' fees or the costs of a judgment.

Unlike state credentialing boards, professional organizations are not immune from lawsuits. By issuing sanctions against MHP members for unethical conduct, professional organizations' ethics committees and the leadership of the professional organization run the risk of being sued by sanctioned MHPs. This issue is important to MHPs as members of these ethics committees because they may be personally liable for their actions. Typically the best protection against liability for serving on one's professional association's ethics committee is liability insurance designed for professional organizational work.

II

MENTAL HEALTH SERVICES RELATED TO INDIVIDUALS, FAMILIES, THE STATE, AND THE WORKPLACE

INTRODUCTION:
MENTAL HEALTH SERVICES RELATED
TO INDIVIDUALS, FAMILIES, THE
STATE, AND THE WORKPLACE

In Part I, we considered issues surrounding the business of mental health services; in this section, we consider the way the law directly affects the delivery of mental health services and in many situations creates new practice opportunities. These services may be for (a) individuals (e.g., evaluating various competencies of individuals, such as the competency to sign a will or manage one's estate), (b) families (e.g., education of children with disabilities), (c) the state (e.g., providing state-mandated services to persons who are mentally ill and dangerous), and (d) the employment sector (e.g., responding to persons claiming sexual harassment in the workplace). The services may occur in a private setting (e.g., therapy in private practice) or a public setting (e.g., services in a state hospital). The services may have nothing to do with a lawsuit (e.g., assessing one's competency to drive), lead to litigation (e.g., therapy for sexual harassment), or arise out of litigation (e.g., assessing a criminal defendant's responsibility at the time of a crime). After reading Part II, one will come to appreciate that the law defines many areas for mental health service.

To exemplify some of these issues, we consider four scenarios:

1. Consider the case of Kim Song who comes to the office of an MHP who sees clients as part of a private practice in a major

metropolitan city. Over the course of meetings, she appears quite distraught and reveals to the MHP a number of concerns about her family. She is worried about her son who is disabled and is getting into trouble at school. What services should he be receiving at school? Who will pay for them? What will happen if he gets arrested? Mrs. Song learned that her daughter is considering having an abortion if her boyfriend does not marry her. Can her daughter get an abortion if she does not approve? Can her daughter get married at her young age? She says her husband intimidates her physically. How can she protect herself? If the MHP learns that she has been beaten, what are his or her responsibilities? What services are available to her as a victim of domestic violence? Mrs. Song also reports that her husband boasts that he will divorce her and win full custody of the children. If the divorce ensues, what is the MHP's role in the proceedings as her therapist? Last, Mrs. Song claims that her husband's mother, who lives with the family, is developing memory and motor problems such that she, Mrs. Song, cannot leave her alone in the house. What can she do to help her mother-in-law? Might she need the aid of the courts? What should she do if she discovers that her mother-in-law is dying? Will the mother-in-law's will be valid given her memory problems?

2. What if an attorney calls and asks an MHP to assist him in an upcoming criminal case? His client has been charged with murdering her husband. The attorney wants to argue that his client was a battered spouse and legally insane at the time of the murder. He also is concerned about her current mental status, believing that she is so impaired that she may not be able to aid him in her defense in the upcoming criminal trial against her. What can an MHP do to help him? Is he or she familiar with the legal standards for competency to stand trial, mens rea, provocation, diminished capacity, and criminal responsibility? Is he or she aware under what conditions battered woman's syndrome may be introduced into a trial?

3. Or consider, for example, a man who rapes a woman. Her attorney may want an MHP to evaluate the woman and testify in the criminal case, and in a subsequent civil case that sues the offender for financial damages. Will he or she be aware of how rape trauma syndrome is relevant to both trials? What if the civil suit is for intentional infliction of emotional distress? Will the MHP know what the legal standard is that he or she will need to address in his or her evaluation and on the witness stand?

4. Finally, consider the problem of a computer wizard named Suzanna Lee who signs a contract with a large software company to develop a new computer game program. However, when working at the company's headquarters, Lee encounters some problems and comes to an MHP for assistance. Not only is she claiming that she has been sexually harassed in her otherwise all-male office but she says that she developed carpal tunnel syndrome while working at the company's computer workstations. Later, she discloses to you that she is afraid of her abusive ex-boyfriend who does not know about her job. She fears that he will assault her at her work if he finds out. Many of the legal questions an MHP might have about this example are addressed in this section (e.g., Can she make a workers compensation claim for her injuries? Does her company need to take steps to protect her and her coworkers from her ex-boyfriend?).

Collectively, the 11 chapters in Part II will help MHPs recognize new practice opportunities, reevaluate the quality of the current services that they are performing in these areas, and give them a better appreciation about why knowledge of the law can enhance their practice as an MHP.

5

COMPETENCY DETERMINATIONS

The law requires that people be competent to engage in certain activities, including: driving, voting, testifying in court, marrying, signing a will, making personal and financial decisions for themselves, and consenting to an abortion as a minor. Mental health professionals (MHPs) may be asked to assist the court in making such competency determinations. MHPs may also be involved in assessments of an individual's competency to enter into a contract, which is discussed in chapter 15.

COMPETENCY TO OBTAIN A DRIVER'S LICENSE

A person who applies for a driver's license must have the requisite mental competency, and thus MHPs may be involved in providing evidence regarding the competency of an applicant. In addition, some states require MHPs to report clients they suspect are unfit to drive. Licenses may be denied, suspended, or revoked for several reasons, including

- adjudication of mental incompetency or incapacitation;
- imposition of a guardianship and conservatorship (see the section titled Conservatorship for Adults in this chap.);

- inability to drive safely because of alcoholism, excessive and chronic use of alcohol or drugs, or addiction to or habitual use of any illegal substance; and
- inability to drive safely because of physical or mental disability or disease (e.g., lapses of consciousness as a result of uncontrolled epilepsy).

In these cases, the state department of motor vehicles (DMV) usually allows applicants to show whether their condition has been compensated for and that they can safely operate a motor vehicle.

Driver's license disqualification may be temporary. For example, a state may regard the person as competent to obtain a license when the person's guardianship is terminated (see the section titled How is a Guardianship Terminated? in this chap.), when the person's mental health is restored, and when the person is released from involuntary civil commitment (see chap. 10). Some states also require that a licensed physician or other proper authority sign a certificate as to the person's condition before the person may apply for a license. Finally, the DMV must make reasonable accommodations to assist otherwise qualified persons with a disability to apply for a driver's license because federal law prohibits discrimination against people with mental and other disabilities.

COMPETENCY TO VOTE

The right to vote may be denied or revoked on the basis of a person's mental impairment or disorder. MHPs may be asked to evaluate people whose competency to vote is at issue. To vote in a state or federal election, a person must first register to vote. At the time of registration, the person may be disqualified from voting if he or she is not able to complete the voter registration form or affidavit and if any of the following mental status issues apply (these vary by state):

1. The person is under a guardianship (see the section titled Guardianship for Adults in this chap.).
2. The person has been found to be *non compos mentis*, insane, or otherwise mentally disabled or incompetent. *Non compos mentis* is a general term for mental disorder but may also be separately defined in one's state's statute. Presumably, these terms refer to a mental disorder or illness that renders a person unable to discharge voting responsibilities.
3. The person has been found not guilty by reason of insanity and is deemed to be gravely disabled (see chap. 13).
4. The person has been found not competent to stand trial and a trial or judgment has been suspended (see chap. 13).

After a person has registered to vote, the county recorder or other government agent must cancel that person's voting registration when there is a legal finding that the person is incompetent or incapacitated or when the person has been civilly committed (see chap. 10). The court in such a case would make a finding that the person has a mental illness or disorder that negates the person's legal responsibility or capacity for carrying out the specific task in question (i.e., voting).

Voting disqualification may be temporary. A state may reinstate voting privileges when the person's guardianship is terminated, when the person's mental health is restored, and when the person is released from involuntary civil commitment. Finally, voting registrars must make reasonable accommodations to assist qualified persons who have a disability to vote because federal law prohibits discrimination against people with mental and other disabilities.

COMPETENCY TO TESTIFY

A witness in a civil or criminal trial must have the requisite mental capacity and the ability to accurately and clearly express him- or herself in court. Any other rule would open the fairness of the trial to question. Thus, a person's ability to testify is determined at the time of the legal proceeding, not at the time that the person witnessed the event.

The issue of competency to testify often arises in cases in which a witness is thought to be too young, mentally ill, or otherwise under sufficient mental distress so as not to be able to testify accurately and truthfully. Whenever questions arise about an adult's or child's competency, MHPs may be asked to provide the court with an assessment of the individual and to testify as to their findings.

What Is the Legal Test of Competency to Testify?

In general, every person regardless of age is qualified to be a witness. A person is only disqualified to testify if it is determined that the person is

- unable to express him- or herself with sufficient clarity (either directly or through an interpreter);
- unable to understand the duty of a witness to tell the truth or understand the nature of an oath;
- mentally impaired or ill such that the person is deprived of the ability to perceive the event about which the person is to testify or is deprived of the ability to recollect and communicate his or her impressions of the facts; and

- because of young age, unable to appreciate the significance of telling the truth or presumed by the law to be incompetent to testify.

A history of drug or alcohol abuse does not by itself make a witness incompetent because it does not, without more information, establish a lack of capacity to fulfill the statutory criteria to testify (e.g., observe, perceive, recollect, and communicate information to the court).

Concern over a witness's ability to testify is not limited to trial testimony. It should also be noted that legal proceedings are not limited to trials. Witnesses are frequently first questioned by the attorneys while under oath at depositions (a pretrial meeting in which witnesses are questioned under oath in the same manner as they would be questioned at trial). If the witness is later unable to testify at trial, then the competency issue will rest on whether the person was competent at the deposition. For instance, one case involved an elderly victim who was incompetent at trial, but her videotaped deposition was admitted after a psychologist testified that she was competent at the time of the taping.

Who Determines One's Competency to Testify?

The determination of whether a witness is competent is within the discretion of the court; it is not a jury matter. The decision process may be broken down into three parts. First, once the competency issue has been raised, the court determines whether it should conduct a preliminary interrogation of the witness. Second, if there is a reasonable doubt regarding the witness's competency, the court determines whether to order an additional examination by an MHP. The court may forgo a mental status examination if it feels that such procedures will not help it make a decision. Finally, on the basis of its own questioning and any evaluations conducted by an MHP, the court determines whether the witness is competent.

COMPETENCY TO MARRY

To marry, many states require that the two people be of a minimum age and mentally competent to consent to the marriage contract. A marriage may be voided or annulled if either person lacked the requisite mental capacity to consent.

Although the test for competency to marry varies between the states, it typically includes showing that at the time of marriage, the party was able to understand the nature of the marriage contract and of the duties and responsibilities it entails and that the party gave free and intelligent consent. MHPs may be called on to evaluate marriage applicants if there is a question about their capacity to consent.

Although the law provides that adults are typically capable of consenting to a marriage, minors will not be allowed to marry unless they have the consent of their parents or guardians or are emancipated under the law. Emancipation means that a minor is deemed by a court to be independent of his or her parents. MHPs may be asked to provide testimony as to the minor's capacity to be emancipated.

Finally, if the person who seeks to marry is competent but a court has doubts about an applicant's ability to fulfill the marriage responsibilities, some states require the judge to consider ordering the parties to participate in premarital counseling concerning the social, economic, and personal responsibilities involved in marriage. This is because in reaching a decision about the marriage application, a judge would also take into consideration the statutory goals of marriage, including reduction of divorce, promotion of child welfare, and/or the best interests of the applicant. MHPs may be involved in such premarital counseling.

COMPETENCY TO SIGN A WILL

Persons who make wills (i.e., testators) or who amend existing ones must meet minimum mental status requirements. If it is shown that the testator does not or did not have the requisite mental capacity at the time of the signing of the will, the estate will be distributed according to the terms of a previous valid will if any or by the state's laws regarding intestacy (i.e., dying without a will).

Mental health consultation or testimony may be used in cases in which an MHP treated or evaluated the testator. Alternatively, MHPs may be asked to provide an opinion of the person's mental status at the time the will was signed based on reports of other witnesses and any other relevant information.

What Is the Test of Testamentary Capacity?

The test of testamentary capacity generally provides that any person may make a will if he or she is (a) 18 or more years of age, is or has been married, or is a member of the military and (b) of sound mind. The test of whether the testator was of sound mind at the time the will was signed requires proof that the testator is or was able to understand

- the nature and extent of his or her property,
- his or her relationships with persons who have a natural claim to the estate property (i.e., family members) and whose interests are affected by the terms of the will,
- the manner of distribution set forth in the will, and

- the consequences of signing the will.

The court determines the issue of whether the testator has or had the capacity to know what he or she is or was doing. Because this decision is based on evidence of the testator's condition at the time the will was signed, testimony by MHPs can be valuable in making such determination.

Courts generally do not like to overturn reasonable wills and are flexible in the amount of mental capacity required to make a will. Thus, although there are several types of mental conditions that may form the basis or part of the basis for a challenge to the will, they do not conclusively prove testamentary incapacity. These conditions include

- mental illness or disorders—on the one hand, symptoms of mental illness will not automatically make a person incompetent to make a will; similarly, adjudication of guardianship (see the section titled Guardianship for Adults in this chap.) will not conclusively fulfill this condition; even adjudicated incompetent people may have lucid intervals during which they meet the sound mind requirements; on the other hand, a mental disorder will invalidate a will if the disorder is of such a broad character as to establish general mental incompetence of the person at the signing of the will or if the symptoms of the disorder (e.g., hallucinations and paranoid ideation) directly affected the dispository provisions of the will;
- mental retardation—courts may still find a person competent to make a will even though the person is mentally retarded and functioning at a mental age below 18 years and even in states where the statute generally requires a testator to be at least 18 years old;
- illiteracy—an illiterate person may make a will if there is other evidence that the person was informed of the contents of the will;
- drug or alcohol abuse—drug or alcohol use by itself will not negate testamentary capacity;
- suicide or attempted suicide—suicide or attempted suicide will not in itself indicate mental incapacity to make a will; and
- senility—senility, mental slowness, poor memory, childishness, eccentricities, and physical infirmities will not by themselves prove a lack of testamentary capacity.

How Are Wills Challenged?

The decedent (i.e., a testator who has died) is presumed to have had testamentary capacity, so people challenge wills by proving either testamentary incapacity or undue influence. The determination of whether the decedent lacked testamentary capacity or was unduly influenced is a factual issue for the jury to decide, if there is one, or for the judge to decide when no jury is present. An MHP's testimony is frequently admitted to argue for or against the capacity of the testator. Note, however, that this is an area in which lay testimony can be equally important in persuading the judge or jury. If an MHP's testimony is contradicted by numerous lay witnesses who observed the testator at the time of the signing of the will, the court can use the lay witness testimony to support its decision. As to the second way of negating a will, proving that the testator's autonomy was so dominated by another person that it was impossible for the testator to resist such an influence, an MHP's testimony about the mental and emotional state of the testator, the person who allegedly exercised the undue influence, and their relationship prior to and at the signing of the will, will be relevant at trial.

GUARDIANSHIP FOR ADULTS

Courts have the power to appoint guardians for individuals who are unable to care for themselves physically or manage their financial affairs and property. Guardians have broad powers; indeed, guardians will control the lives of their wards much as parents oversee the lives of their children. Guardianship may be obtained for generally two classes of people: minors and incapacitated persons (including those found to be gravely disabled). In this chapter, we discuss guardianships for incapacitated persons (guardianship for minors is discussed in chap. 6). MHPs may become involved in the guardianship process by being asked to evaluate the person who is the subject of a guardianship petition and testify as to whether the person meets the test for guardianship or by providing therapeutic services to the ward after a guardianship has been imposed.

What Is the Legal Standard for Imposing a Guardianship?

For a guardianship to be imposed, the court generally needs to find that the person is incapacitated and that the appointment is necessary or desirable as a means of providing continuing care and supervision of the incapacitated person. The legal standard for incapacitation varies by state but usually means that the person is impaired by reason of mental illness, mental disorder, mental retardation, physical illness or disability, advanced age, or chronic use of drugs or alcohol such that the person lacks sufficient understanding or capacity to make or communicate responsible decisions concerning him- or herself.

What Is the Guardianship Process for Incapacitated People?

An incapacitated person or anyone interested in the person's welfare may petition the court for a finding of legal incapacity or mental incompetency and the appointment of a guardian. The law of some states specifically defines who may seek appointment of a guardian for individuals with certain conditions (e.g., mental illness, mental retardation, excessive spending, and physical incapacitation or illness). Some states require the petition to contain certain information, such as the names and addresses of the applicant, the individual requiring the guardianship, the reason for the need for a guardianship, and the proposed guardian.

On receiving the petition, the court must appoint counsel or a guardian *ad litem* (i.e., someone who represents the ward's specific interests in the guardianship hearing) to represent the individual whose capacity is in question. MHPs may serve as guardians *ad litem*. Other requirements may be imposed by one's state at this stage in the process. For example, a common requirement is that a physician and/or MHP examine the allegedly incapacitated person, and submit a written report to the court.

At the guardianship hearing, the allegedly incapacitated person may have the following rights, including to be present and hear all the evidence; be represented by counsel; cross-examine all witnesses, including the physician and MHP; have a trial by jury; and have the matter decided at a closed hearing.

Who May Be Appointed as a Guardian?

As a general rule, any competent person may be appointed as guardian. The law in some states, however, specifies who may serve as a guardian. Some states require that the choice of guardian be made according to a list of priorities. For example, the law of one state provides that priority be given to the following individuals:

- the spouse of the incapacitated person;
- an adult child of the incapacitated person;
- a parent of the incapacitated person, including a person nominated by will or other writing signed by a deceased parent;
- any relative of the incapacitated person with whom that person has resided for more than 6 months prior to the filing of the petition; and
- the nominee of a person who is caring for or paying benefits to the incapacitated person.

What Is the Authority of a Guardian?

The authority of the guardian will vary depending on whether the state has a plenary or limited guardianship approach. Under a plenary guardianship statute, guardians of incapacitated persons generally have the same powers, rights, and duties concerning their wards that parents have over unemancipated minors. However, the guardian is not legally responsible to provide for the ward out of his or her own funds or liable for the acts of the ward. State law may also provide for some of the following powers and duties of a guardian:

- to have custody of the ward and establish the ward's residence in or out of the state;
- to provide for the ward's care, comfort, and welfare;
- to provide for the training and education of the ward;
- to take reasonable care of the ward's clothing, furniture, vehicles, and personal property;
- to consent to medical or other professional treatment of the ward, or if it cannot be provided, to institute proceedings to compel persons under a duty to support the ward to pay the required sums;
- to receive money and tangible property deliverable to the ward if no conservator has been appointed (see the section titled Conservatorship for Adults in this chap.);
- to receive money for support of the ward's care and education;
- to protect the ward's freedom of religion and religious practice; and
- to report on the condition of the ward as specified by court order.

In limited guardianship states, the powers of the guardian will be limited to only those areas of incapacity that can be behaviorally specified and proven. MHPs may be asked by guardians

- for advice and assistance in determining the needs of the ward,
- to evaluate the ward periodically,
- to provide treatment that offers the best opportunity to achieve recovery from the mental illness and disability, and
- to suggest alternatives to hospitalization for the ward.

Persons who have been declared incompetent may sue or defend against a lawsuit through their guardian. The guardian does not assume any liability but will direct the conduct of the case for the incompetent person. If the person has not had a guardian appointed, the court may appoint a guardian *ad litem* to stand in for the person during the legal proceeding.

How Is a Guardianship Terminated?

The authority and responsibility of a guardian generally terminates if

- the ward dies,
- the guardian dies,

- a court determines that the guardian is incapacitated,
- a court removes the guardian,
- the guardian resigns, or
- the court finds that the ward's competency has been restored.

CONSERVATORSHIP FOR ADULTS

In some states, as previously noted, a guardian is appointed to manage both the personal affairs and the financial affairs (including property) of the ward. In other states, a guardian is appointed to manage the ward's personal affairs, and a conservator is appointed to manage the estate (e.g., property, financial resources, and business enterprises) of a minor or an adult who is no longer able to manage his or her property and/or financial affairs. And finally, at least in one state the conservator is appointed to manage both the personal affairs and the financial affairs (including property) of the ward. If a guardian or conservator can manage all affairs of the ward, the other type of substitute decision maker is not recognized under the law.

If states have both guardianship and conservatorship, the latter provides a more limited form of supervision because a conservator only has power over the person's property—not his or her person. This allows wards of conservators to be able to make their own personal decisions, including health care, choice of living arrangement, and other matters. In this section, we cover conservatorship for adults (conservatorship for minors is discussed in chap. 6).

MHPs may become involved in this process by being asked to evaluate the person and to testify as to the person's capacity to manage his or her estate. MHPs may also provide therapeutic services to the person after a conservatorship has been imposed.

What Is the Legal Standard for Imposing a Conservatorship?

Before a conservator may be appointed, the court must determine that the person meets the legal standards for appointment of a conservator. In general, this involves a finding that there is an underlying basis for the person's inability to manage his or her property or estate. The basis (e.g., mental illness, mental disorder, mental incompetence, physical illness, advanced age, chronic use of drugs or alcohol, confinement, detention by a foreign power, or the person's disappearance) is usually specified in state law. If a person is receiving Veterans Administration (VA) benefits and has been found incapable of handling the benefits, the VA examination may constitute proof of the necessity for conservatorship. In reaching its judgment, the court may direct the person to be examined by a physician and/or MHP.

Who May Seek an Application for Conservatorship?

In general, any person, including the one to be protected, may petition the court for the appointment of a conservator. This includes those who would be adversely affected by lack of effective management of the property and affairs of the proposed ward as well as those interested in the person's well-being. Some states, however, specifically restrict the persons who are allowed to apply for the conservatorship of another person.

What Is Involved in the Conservatorship Application Process?

The petition for conservatorship is filed with the court. State law may have requirements that the petition must follow, such as describing

- the interest of the petitioner;
- the name, age, residence, and address of the proposed ward;
- the name and address of the guardian if any has been appointed;
- the name and address of the nearest relative of the proposed ward;
- the names and addresses of the heirs of the proposed ward;
- a general statement of the property of the proposed ward with an estimate of its value, including any compensation, insurance, pension, or allowance to which the person is entitled;
- reasons why appointment of a conservator is necessary; and
- reasons for the appointment of a particular person or entity (e.g., a bank) as conservator.

After receiving a petition, the court will set a date for the hearing. The person as well as others (such as the person's spouse, heirs, and parents) must then be personally served with notice of the hearing within a certain time (e.g., 14 days) before the hearing. Unless the person has an attorney, the court must appoint one or a guardian *ad litem* who will advocate for the person's best interests.

Who May Serve as a Conservator?

The court may appoint an individual or corporation (e.g., a qualified financial institution) as conservator of the person's estate. In addition, state law may specify an order of preference, which the court may bypass with good reason. For example, one state provides for the following order of preference for a conservator:

- a person who regularly acts as conservator in that jurisdiction,
- an individual or corporation nominated by the protected person,

- the spouse of the protected person,
- an adult child of the protected person,
- a relative of the protected person with whom that person has lived for more than six months prior to the filing of the petition, and
- the nominee of a person who is caring for or paying benefits to the protected person.

What Are the Authority and Responsibilities of the Conservator?

The duties of a conservator generally include handling the ward's financial affairs, managing the ward's estate for the benefit of the ward, and initiating or responding to any legal actions concerning debts owed to or by the ward. The conservator is generally held to a standard that would be observed by a prudent person handling the financial affairs of another. Some states require special court authorization for significant decisions (e.g., selling real estate, making substantial gifts, and dispersing assets for tax purposes).

How Is the Conservatorship Terminated?

Any interested person, including the ward, may petition the court to terminate the conservatorship. A conservatorship may also be terminated by the death of the ward or conservator or if the conservator was found to be mentally incompetent. On termination of the conservatorship, the ward fully controls his or her property and financial affairs.

MINORS' COMPETENCY TO CONSENT TO AN ABORTION

Although it is constitutionally forbidden for the state to impose regulations that would give parents a veto power over a minor woman's right to an abortion, the state may impose a parental notification requirement. Not all states have enacted such parental notification laws.

MHPs may become involved in this process by evaluating and testifying as to whether the minor woman is mature enough to make the decision to have an abortion without parental notification, the likely impact of parental notification on the minor, and whether notification would be against her best interests.

What Is Parental Notification Law?

These laws generally provide that a physician may not perform an abortion on an unemancipated minor woman unless a parent or legal guardian is first notified that she intends to obtain an abortion. Written consent of the parent or guardian may also be required. However, notification is not required when the minor woman receives a judicial order that she is mature enough to make the abortion decision or that her best interests would be served even if she is immature by obtaining an abortion without parental notification.

Some states have provided for other exceptions to the notification requirement, such as

- a parent or legal guardian cannot be located and the treating physician or the woman certifies in writing the efforts made to notify the parents or
- there is an emergency need for an abortion to be performed such that continuation of the pregnancy is an immediate threat and grave risk to the life of the pregnant woman, and the attending physician certifies that fact in writing.

May an Incompetent Woman Obtain an Abortion?

Although not all states have addressed this issue, a court may approve a petition for an abortion brought on behalf of a woman found to be incompetent. In making this determination, the court will determine whether the person has the capacity to make such a decision. If the person is not found to have such capacity, the court will typically appoint a guardian *ad litem* to make the decision for the women. Depending on state law, such substituted judgments are based either on whether the person, if competent, would have elected to have the abortion or on whether the abortion is in the incompetent person's best interests. In some cases, the court will decide to make the decision itself without appointing a guardian *ad litem* to represent the woman's interests before the court. Expert testimony about the woman by MHPs may be relevant in such determinations.

6

CHILD CARE AND PROTECTION

The court may ask mental health professionals (MHPs) to assist in making decisions about the welfare and placement of children in guardianship, conservatorship, foster care, adoption, and abuse and neglect cases. MHPs need to know the law in this area because state law may affect their assessments in these cases.

GUARDIANSHIP FOR MINORS

A guardian may be appointed for a minor in situations in which the custodial parent(s) is (are) unable to care for the child as a result of death, legal termination of parental rights, mental illness, or other circumstances. In some states, guardians are appointed to undertake parental responsibilities, and conservators (see the section titled Conservatorship for Minors in this chap.) are appointed to manage the minor's estate (e.g., money, property, and business enterprises). States that do not distinguish between guardians and conservators include estate management within their guardianship law. Finally, at least one state refers to both guardians and conservators as conservators.

MHPs are likely to become involved in the guardianship process by testifying about their evaluation as to whether the child is at risk unless a guardianship is created and whether someone being considered for appointment as the guardian will present any psychological problems for the child. In addition, MHPs may provide the child's follow-up assessment and treatment at the request of the guardian.

What Is the Process for Appointing a Guardian for a Minor?

There are two possible methods for appointing a guardian for a minor: testamentary appointment and petitioning the court. In testamentary appointment, parents, in anticipation of death, may indicate in their will whom they wish to be guardian of their children. Some states allow for testamentary appointments to be made for children who are in utero. Testamentary appointments are valuable when both parents die or otherwise become totally incapacitated while their children are still minors.

In general, a testamentary appointment becomes effective when the guardian files an acceptance in the court in which the will is probated. Probate refers to the process whereby a court oversees the administration and distribution of a deceased person's estate. Other individuals may challenge the new appointment in court. Some states specify who may bring such an action. One state, for example, allows anyone to inquire into the custody of the minor and empowers the court to alter the testamentary guardianship to conform to the child's best interests. In another state, children over 13 may object to a testamentary appointment by filing a written objection in the probate court before the estate is settled or within 30 days after the court is notified of the guardian's acceptance. If the child objects, the court will schedule a guardianship hearing and make the appointment; however, the court may appoint the person named in the testamentary appointment notwithstanding the child's objection.

In petitioning the court, a person or entity (e.g., Child Protection Services [CPS]) may allege that a minor is in need of a guardianship because of

- being abandoned,
- being abused or neglected,
- being developmentally disabled such that the child's needs cannot be met at home, or
- death of the parents who have not made a testamentary appointment.

Who May Serve as the Guardian?

If the court determines that a guardianship is warranted, the court will determine who should be appointed guardian. In considering a given candidate, the court generally determines whether the appointment would be in the best interests of the minor. Unfortunately, many states do not have law highlighting important factors for the court to use in reaching its decision. Some states allow minors above a certain age (e.g., 12 years) to select the guardian, subject to court approval. Other states specify who may not serve as a guardian (e.g., minors, incapacitated persons, or persons who lack education or experience to manage either the property or the minor).

What Are the Powers and Duties of a Minor's Guardian?

In general, guardians of minors have the same powers and responsibilities of parents, except that guardians are not legally obligated to provide their own funds for children and may not be liable to third parties for the acts of the children. State law may further specify other duties and responsibilities of the guardian, such as to

- take reasonable care of the child's personal effects;
- receive money payable for the support of the child;
- exercise care to conserve any excess funds for the child's future needs;
- facilitate the child's education and social and other activities;
- provide authorization for the child's medical or other professional care, treatment, or advice;
- consent to the marriage or adoption of the child; and
- report to the court on the child's condition if required to do so by the court's guardianship order.

Despite the guardian's powers, the court retains final authority over the ward (i.e., the minor child who has been given a guardian).

How Is the Guardianship Terminated?

Any person interested in the child's welfare may petition for removal of the guardian on the ground that removal would be in the best interests of the child. The court then has a hearing to determine whether it is in the child's best interests to terminate the guardianship. If it is, then the court will appoint a new guardian. A guardian's authority and responsibility also will be terminated on the death or resignation of the guardian; on the child's death, adoption, or marriage; or when the child reaches 18.

CONSERVATORSHIP FOR MINORS

In some states, guardians are appointed to undertake parental responsibilities for minors when the parents are absent or incapacitated (see previous sections), whereas conservators are charged with the responsibilities of managing or protecting the minor's estate (e.g., money, property, and business enterprises). There is no requirement that the minor also have a guardian appointed. As already noted in the section titled Guardianship for Minors, in states that do not have a distinction between guardians and conservators, management of the estate is covered under guardianship law. Finally, at least one state refers to both guardians and conservators as conservators (see the previous section titled Guardianship for Minors).

MHPs are less likely to become involved in the conservatorship process than in the guardianship process. If they do become involved, they may be asked to testify about their evaluation as to whether the child is at risk unless a conservatorship is created and whether someone being considered for appointment as the conservator will present any psychological problems for the child.

What Is the Process for Appointing a Conservator for Minors?

Any person, including the minor to be protected, may petition the court for the appointment of a conservator. This includes those who would be adversely affected by the lack of effective management of the minor's property and affairs as well as those interested in the minor's well-being. The contents of the petition will vary by state but generally will describe

- the interest of the petitioner (the person bringing the petition before the court);
- the name, age, residence, and address of the minor;
- the name and address of the minor's guardian, if there is one;
- the name and address of the nearest relative of the minor who is known to the petitioner;
- a general statement of the property of the person to be protected with an estimate of its value, including any compensation, insurance, pension, or allowance that is due to the minor;
- reasons why appointment of a conservator is necessary; and
- reasons why the court should appoint a particular person or entity (e.g., a bank) as conservator.

If at any time in the conservatorship proceeding, the court determines that the interest of the minor may be inadequately represented, it may appoint an attorney to represent the minor with or without a guardian *ad litem*. In some states, the court must give consideration to the minor's preference for a particular attorney if the child is over a certain age (e.g., 13 years).

Generally, the court may appoint a conservator if it determines that the minor owns money, property, or interest in a business that requires management or protection by a conservator or funds are needed for the support and education of the minor and the appointment of a conservator is desirable to satisfy these needs.

Note that these circumstances are broad enough to include situations in which a conservator may be appointed even though the parents are present and fulfilling the other parental duties. This is especially true if a third party has injured the minor and a lawsuit has been filed to obtain a monetary award for the child's damages. It may not be possible to settle the lawsuit without the appointment of a conservator.

Who May Serve as the Conservator?

The court may appoint an individual or an entity as conservator of the minor's estate. Some states indicate an order of preference for appointing conservators. The law of one state, for example, provides the following order of preference, which the court may bypass with good reason:

- a person who regularly acts as conservator in that jurisdiction,
- an individual or entity nominated by the minor if the child is over 13,
- a relative of the minor with whom the child has lived for more than 6 months prior to the filing of the petition, and
- the nominee of a person who is caring for the protected minor or paying benefits to the minor.

What Are the Powers of the Conservator?

The authority of the conservator may be very broad, including selling, transferring, dividing, or otherwise managing the minor's property and financial holdings for the benefit of the minor. The conservator is generally held to a standard that would be observed by a prudent person handling the financial affairs of another. However, some states require special court authorization for such decisions (e.g., selling real estate, making substantial gifts, and dispersing assets for tax purposes).

How Is the Conservatorship Terminated?

Any interested person, including the conservatee, may petition the court to terminate the conservatorship. A conservatorship may also be terminated by the death of the minor or on a finding of mental incompetency of the conservator.

FOSTER CARE

Foster care provides 24-hour-per-day housing and substitute care for children (and adults in some states) who are not able to live in their home because their family cannot or will not provide normal family care for them. The person may be placed in a foster home for as little as one night or as long as several years. Foster homes may be single-family homes, group homes, or larger child-care institutions. MHPs may be involved in licensing foster homes, evaluating prospective foster parents for suitability, training foster family licensees, and providing assessment and therapeutic services to those persons placed in foster care.

What Are Licensing Requirements for Foster Care?

In some states, foster parent applicants must be licensed. Other states require that applicants and their homes meet detailed standards. The application process generally includes completing a series of forms, undergoing background checks and home visits, engaging in specialized training, and being interviewed by state appointed professionals, including MHPs.

Foster parents

- usually are over the age of 21 but must be at least 18 if the spouse or partner is at least 21 years old;
- may be single, married, divorced, separated, widowed, or cohabiting, but some states' policies favor traditional families and disfavor nontraditional families, such as homosexual couples;
- may be of any religion or have no religion, as long as the religious practices do not interfere with the foster child's receiving medical care;
- must undergo a fingerprint or other criminal record check;
- must have no history of, and present no risk of, abuse or neglect;
- must have income independent of foster care payments such that the foster parents do not rely on the payments made for the persons in their care; provide a work phone number where the applicant can be reached in case of an emergency; and have acceptable child care provisions established if both applicants are employed outside the home; and
- must be in good physical and mental health and free from any emotional problems or substance abuse that would prevent them from properly caring for foster children.

Foster parents must show ability to

- provide nurturance, warmth, and intellectual stimulation to the child;
- protect the child from harm;
- appropriately respond to the child's emotional, social, physical, developmental, cultural, ethnic, educational, and intellectual needs;

- not use corporal or emotionally damaging discipline;
- cooperate with any activities in the foster child's case plan, including providing services by MHPs;
- provide the child with his or her own bed in a room with adequate space for his or her belongings;
- maintain the home in a safe and sanitary manner; and
- be willing to participate in specialized training when offered by the state agency responsible for overseeing foster care placements.

The state agency generally provides for the medical, dental, and mental health care for all children in foster care.

In addition to these requirements, a foster home may qualify to receive children with special cultural, ethnic, physical, emotional, or behavioral needs or background. Parents in these special foster homes must have had previous training or experience or demonstrate a willingness to care for children with special needs. They must also have the ability to work effectively with specialists involved in the evaluation and treatment of the child.

A foster home may also qualify to provide short-term emergency foster care. These foster homes must be exceptionally flexible and capable of accepting children of varied cultural and racial backgrounds and be able to handle emotional stress at all hours of the day and night.

What Are Requirements for Placement in a Foster Home?

Prior to placement of a person in a foster home, the state agency or a licensed child welfare agency may arrange for a complete medical or other examination to evaluate and if necessary diagnose the child who is to be placed. If the examination discloses no reasons for special care, the child may be placed in a regular foster home. If special care is required, the child may be placed only in a foster home that is certified as a special foster home.

After placement of the person in foster care, some states require the agency responsible for these placements to document for the court that placement was in the child's best interests and that reasonable efforts were made to avoid the placement. In addition, the agency usually must establish a placement plan that is submitted directly to either the court or the state's foster care placement review board. The placement plan may contain

- the purpose for which the child has been placed in foster care,
- the length of time in which the purpose of foster care will be accomplished,
- the description of the services that are to be provided in order for the purpose of foster care to be accomplished, and
- the name of the person in the agency responsible for foster care placements who is directly responsible for assuring that the plan is implemented.

When the court reviews the foster care placement, it will use the best interests of the child and the least restrictive setting or placement as standards to guide its decision. Some states also require review boards and courts to give priority to returning the child to the natural parents during the 1st year of placement. After a year in foster care, the priority shifts to finding an alternate permanent placement with a relative or through adoption. Other states allow for long-term foster care when neither reuniting the child with natural parents nor adoption is in the child's best interests.

ADOPTION

The purpose of adoption is to provide stable homes for children while at the same time attempting as much as possible to protect the rights of the child, the biological parents, and the adoptive parents. Adoption may be a voluntary process in which parental rights are relinquished or an involuntary process in which parental rights are terminated.

MHPs may be asked to evaluate and testify about the mental status of children subject to adoption, the qualifications of potential adoptive parents, and/or postplacement evaluations. If necessary, they may also provide treatment to the adopted children. Some states specifically provide for the state agency that conducts the investigation to contract for mental health evaluations of the child and include them in the report.

Who May Be Adopted?

Generally, only children who are under the age of 18 at the time a petition for adoption is filed may be adopted. Some states also specifically require the consent of a child who is above a certain age (e.g., 12 years old) before he or she can be adopted.

An evaluation of the child must be made before the child is placed for adoption. Conducted by an officer of the court, agency, or other governmental agency, the investigation and resulting written report should include certain information, such as

- whether the natural parents, if living, are willing to have the child be adopted and the reasons for such willingness;
- whether the natural parents have abandoned the child or are unfit to have custody of the child;
- whether the parent–child relationship has been previously terminated by court action and the circumstances of the termination;
- the racial, ethnic, and religious background of the child and the natural parents;

- the mental and physical condition of the child and natural parents (taken from medical reports, genetic history, psychological evaluations, and academic information about the child);
- the child's developmental and social history and family life, including information on prior placements;
- the existing and proposed arrangements as to the custody of the child, including advisability of placing the child with siblings;
- the adoptability of the child; and
- the suitability of the child's placement with the applicants.

What Are the Requirements to Be Adoptive Parents?

As a general rule, any legally competent adult resident of a state, whether married, unmarried, or legally separated may try to qualify to adopt children. A husband and wife may jointly adopt children. Some states specifically allow same-sex couples to be adoptive families. A state may specify a minimum age (e.g., 18 years) or other age requirement (e.g., at least 10 years older than the child to be adopted), or consider the life expectancy of the prospective parent(s).

The evaluation of prospective adoptive parents is referred to as preadoption certification in some states. This evaluation might be conducted by a staff member of the presiding court, the state agency responsible for overseeing adoptions, or another government agency (e.g., the department of social services or CPS), with the results being submitted to the presiding court or agency. The investigation and resulting report generally contains a complete social history of the applicants and information about their financial condition, moral fitness, religious background, physical and mental condition, and criminal background, including any court actions involving child abuse. Some states require the prospective adoptive parents to submit their fingerprints as part of the criminal background check, and the resulting criminal record is then assessed for its effects on the ability of the parent to provide adequate care and guidance to the child.

In states that require preadoption certification, the court certifies the applicants as being acceptable or unacceptable to adopt children on the basis of the findings and recommendations of the report. The certification remains in effect for 1 year and may be extended for an unlimited number of 1-year periods if, after review, the court finds that there have been no material changes in circumstances that would affect the acceptability of the applicants to adopt. Any applicant who has been certified as nonacceptable may petition the court for review. The matter will be heard by the court, which may affirm or reverse the certification. Nonacceptable candidates may not reapply for certification for 1 year thereafter.

What Is the Process for Adoption?

Persons wishing to adopt a child must petition the court for approval of their application for adoption of a particular child. Before the court can issue an order or final decree of adoption for that child, the adoptive parents will undergo an application and evaluation process that differs by state.

Adoption petitions to a court (see the next section) may take place either independently or through an agency. In an independent adoption, the birth parent personally selects the prospective adoptive parents. Some states require that the selection be based on the birth parents' personal knowledge of the prospective adoptive parent(s). In addition, the proposed independent adoption may be subject to an investigation and approval by a state-approved adoption agency, state department of social services, or other state approved entity or individual.

Agency adoptions involve an agency licensed or approved to place children for adoption in a state that is a party to or joins in the petition for adoption. Agencies generally assess the prospective adoptive parents and match children with assessed and approved prospective applicants. In addition, some full-service adoptive agencies assume the care, custody, and control of a child through either involuntary termination of parental rights or parental relinquishment of their minor to the agency. Some states provide for a supervision period between placement and final adoption of the child. Counseling is often an integral part of this interim process.

What Is Involved in the Adoption Petition and Hearing?

Some states place restrictions on who may file a petition and when the hearing is held on the petition. For example, one state only allows preapproved adoptive parents to file a petition on a child who has been in the care of a state adoption or social services agency. Stepparent adoptions may also be subject to the investigation and petition process. In another state, the hearing on the petition cannot be held until at least 6 months after the petition has been filed.

After the petition has been filed, consent that is deliberate, intentional, and voluntary must be obtained from the appropriate parties for the adoption. The required parties generally include the biological parents (or the legal guardian of the child) as well as the child who is above a certain age (e.g., 14 years). However, consent from the biological parents may not be required in the following circumstances:

- a parent has been declared incompetent (see chap. 5);
- the parental rights have been judicially terminated (see the next section); or
- a court, after a full hearing on the issue, waived the consent requirement because waiver promoted the child's interest.

Historically, the courts have been reluctant to revoke consent after the child has been placed in the adoptive home. However, consent may be revoked if fraud or duress occurred or if the consenting party lacked mental competency at the time of the consent.

In addition, if the court wishes more information, it may direct that the state department responsible for adoptions, an agency, or other qualified personnel (as determined by the court) make an additional social study. As a supplement to the precertification or investigatory report previously discussed, the social study would include information regarding the

- child's social history,
- child's present condition,
- child's present placement and adjustment in the home of the people seeking to become adoptive parents (if any), and
- suitability of the adoptive parents and their home.

An order of adoption will be issued if it is in the best interests of the child. Courts may issue certificates of adoption that may not include the names of the child's biological parents. However, certain information, such as medical reports, may be given to the adoptive parents and child. Adoption orders can also regulate contact between birth parents and the adopted child as well as the release of personal types of information (e.g., letters, photographs, and personal property).

What Is the Legal Effect of Adoption?

After an adoption has been ordered, the biological parent is divested of all legal rights and obligations with regard to the child. The adopted child becomes the child and legal heir of the adoptive parent. An adoptive parent may in some states petition the court to undo an adoption, but such petitions are rarely granted. Petitioners must demonstrate that the adoption agency or other person or entity used fraud or deceit to induce them to enter into the adoption.

What Are Adoption Subsidies?

Some states provide for adoption subsidy programs. Such programs provide monetary assistance and special services for children who otherwise may not be adopted, making it possible to secure adoptive homes with people who meet all but the financial standards for adoptive parents. Generally, children in these programs must be either emotionally attached to the prospective adoptive parents after being in their care as foster children or unlikely to be adopted because of physical or mental disability, emotional disturbance, high risk of physical or mental illness, age, sibling relationship, or racial or ethnic factors. The results of an MHP evaluation usually will determine what services are necessary under the subsidy program.

What Is the Law Regarding Surrogacy?

A surrogacy agreement is a contract in which a woman agrees to be impregnated with the semen of another woman's husband. After the child's birth, the surrogate surrenders the child to the biological father and his wife. Gestational surrogacy refers to the situation in which the husband's sperm is first artificially joined with his wife's egg. The embryo is then implanted in the surrogate, who carries the child. Not all states permit contracts for surrogate children. In one state that allows surrogate arrangements, gestational surrogacy is distinguished from adoption so that it is not subject to the adoption laws.

Because surrogacy agreements usually constitute a contract between private parties (although surrogacy brokers are sometimes involved), the need for a mental health evaluation typically does not arise. It may, however, if the biological parent or parents wish to determine the mental and emotional stability of the surrogate or if one of the parties seeks counseling during the pregnancy or after the birth of the child.

ABUSED AND NEGLECTED CHILDREN

There are several ways in which MHPs may become involved with abused and neglected children. If MHPs suspect abuse, they have a duty to report the suspected abuse or neglect (see chap. 3). Once the abuse has been reported (by either an MHP or another person) to the appropriate agency(ies), procedures for handing child abuse and neglect cases typically involve four stages: investigation, taking the child into temporary custody, holding a hearing on a dependency petition, and holding a hearing on an appropriate disposition. This hierarchical process may stop at any point if the allegations are unfounded or unsupported or if the parents show they are capable of raising their children in a responsible manner. Each stage may involve a mental health evaluation of the child and or parent(s). In addition, the MHP may be called to testify as an expert witness. Finally, MHPs are frequently involved in providing services to abused and neglected children, their families, and other nonfamilial abusers of the child.

What Is the Investigation Process?

Reports of suspected child abuse or neglect (including those made by MHPs) are made to the appropriate agency(ies) as dictated by state law and local governmental policies. Although most states require the report to be made to CPS, a growing number of states use a multi- or interdisciplinary team (MDT or IDT) model that allows reports to be made either to CPS or to law enforcement. Such an approach ensures that the agency to which the report has been made will share the information with the other agency. In addition, law enforcement and CPS collaborate during the investigation process and meet with a broader multidisciplinary team to discuss the next step in the case, if any.

Once CPS or law enforcement receives a report of suspected abuse, the report is screened to determine whether there is reasonable cause to believe that the child was abused or neglected. This process involves gathering as much information as possible about the child, his or her environment, the child's family and other significant people, and the alleged perpetrator(s). At some point in the investigation, all children who have been reported as having been abused or neglected will be seen and interviewed. The investigative interview may be performed by the CPS worker or law enforcement officer assigned to the case. The trend in these cases, however, is to have the child interviewed by a trained forensic interviewer who often is an MHP. Because these interviews are simultaneously observed by members of the MDT and recorded on videotape, the number of interviews of the child is minimized and the quality, reliability, and amount of information obtained about the child is maximized.

The screening or investigatory evaluation ends with a determination by CPS and by law enforcement that the report is either supported and substantiated or screened out as unsupported and unsubstantiated. If the former is found, some states require an MDT conference to determine whether a case will be handled criminally or as a child protective matter. In some states, certain cases proceed directly to prosecution because the district attorney will have to be notified under state law if the case involves death, sexual abuse or exploitation, or severe bodily injury.

When a case is supported, CPS will offer services to the child and family. The child may also be taken into temporary custody (see the next section). CPS or an MHP may also file a petition in civil court for the child's care and protection. In these cases, the court is asked to determine whether the child has been abused or neglected and to authorize services to the child or family. The judge may order appropriate services and may transfer custody of the child to another person or entity in extreme cases. In cases in which a report is not supported but it appears that the family could benefit from services, CPS may offer voluntary services to the family; these could include counseling, parenting classes, day care, homemaker, and chore services. The family is free to accept or reject the services, and the parent may also choose to place the child in foster care. For law enforcement, a supported case may result in taking the child into temporary custody, the arrest of the alleged abuser, and the prosecution of that person.

What Is Temporary Custody?

A law enforcement officer, CPS worker, or other approved individual (e.g., a probation officer or physician) may take a child into temporary custody without a court order for a short period of time (e.g., up to 72 hours) if certain criteria are met. These criteria may include a showing of probable cause to believe that the child has been abused or neglected, that the child is suffering from serious physical or emotional damage, or that the child may be injured or disappear before the court order can be obtained. When taken into custody, the child is placed in the care of the appropriate state agency or a community service program or shelter for abused or neglected children and may receive routine or emergency medical exams and treatment as well as an evaluation of his or her emotional condition. MHPs evaluate the child for symptoms of serious emotional damage, which may include severe anxiety, depression, withdrawal or excessive aggressive behavior toward self or others. State law may also require that the child be permitted to call his or her parents and/or an attorney.

The state agent is required to give the parents or guardians notice that their child has been taken into temporary custody and advise them of their rights in any upcoming legal action. However, in some states, the court may issue an order that the parents or guardians not be notified of the child's exact location if it would put the child and her or his temporary caregivers in danger or if the parent might try to flee with the child.

In cases in which the child has been removed from the home without a court order, many states require that a preliminary hearing (also referred to as detention hearing or temporary custody hearing) be held on the next court day. At that time, the court determines whether the child's interests require continued protection before a full dispositional hearing is held. If so, the court may continue the temporary custodial arrangement and appoint a temporary guardian or conservator (see previous sections in this chap.). If the court finds that the parents do not present a danger to the child, it will return the child to the custody of his or her parents or guardian.

What Is a Dependency Hearing?

A dependency hearing is initiated by the state by filing of a petition with the court based on facts presented by CPS and members of the MDT. At the hearing in a case of child abuse or neglect, the state must prove that the child's circumstances meet the state's legal standards of child abuse or neglect. MHPs may participate as expert witnesses at this and subsequent hearings. The child may also be required to have an attorney and a guardian *ad litem* appointed for him or her to represent the child's best interests.

After the court determines whether the child has been abused or neglected, the court makes written findings of fact concerning the dependency and decides the appropriate temporary placement for the child. At specific intervals (e.g., every 6 months), the court will hold interim hearings and require CPS to show that although they tried to offer the family services to reunify the family, return of custody to the parents would be detrimental to the safety and well-being of the child. The testimony of MHPs is often essential in these cases.

What Are the Dispositional Alternatives?

If the court finds that the allegations in the dependency petition have been proven, a final dispositional hearing is held. At this hearing, the court may consider a social or predispositional study that reviews all of the information pertinent to the case and do one of the following:

- suspend judgment for a period of time (e.g., 1 year), while ordering the parents or guardian to comply with terms and conditions that the court may impose;
- release the child to the custody of the parents or guardian for a period of time (e.g., 1 year) under an order that may include supervision by CPS and other conditions;
- remove the child from the home and place the child in the custody of a suitable institution, an association willing to receive the child, a reputable citizen of good moral character, an appropriate public or private agency licensed to care for children, a foster home in which the child has been placed before an interruption in foster care, a suitable school, or maternal or paternal relatives provided that they are physically and financially able to provide proper care;
- issue a protection order requiring that the parents or guardian follow certain behavioral guidelines, such as staying away from the child or home, avoiding offensive conduct, and permitting child visitation at certain times only;
- place the parent or guardian under the supervision of the state's department of probation;
- require that an individual found to have abused or neglected a child participate in therapeutic services, including psychotherapy, group self-help programs, and functional education;
- require that the child be given therapeutic services to evaluate and treat any damage the child may have suffered; or
- conclude that the child was abandoned by his or her parents or guardian and award custody of the child to CPS.

Ultimately, the court may initiate a hearing to terminate the parent–child relationship. Any person or agency that has a legitimate interest in the parent–child relationship may make that request (see the next section), or the natural parents may voluntarily relinquish custody and care of the child.

TERMINATION OF PARENTAL RIGHTS

After a case of child abuse or neglect has been reported and after it has been substantiated by CPS and/or law enforcement, and usually after the child has been found dependent (see the previous section), the question may arise as to whether parental rights should be terminated. This is an extreme measure reflecting serious family dysfunction. Because such a decision involves consideration of the child's emotional well-being, the parents' functioning, and the parent–child relationship, MHPs are frequently called on to undertake individual and family evaluations to assist the court in deciding whether the parents are fit to retain their children. MHPs may also be involved in providing services to the child before, during, and after this process.

What Is Involved in a Petition for Termination?

Any person, agency, or corporation that has a legitimate interest in the welfare of the child may file a petition for the termination of the parent–child relationship. This includes MHPs working with the child as well as relatives or other interested persons. The court may also initiate such a proceeding.

The contents of the petition, which will vary by state, generally should show why termination of parental rights is in the best interests of the child and how the parent has failed to perform his or her responsibilities or is unfit. Thus, the petition usually contains an assertion that the parent has relinquished rights to the child or that

- the parent is unable to care for the child because of unavailability, which may be a result of abandonment;
- the parent has neglected or willfully abused the child;
- the parent is unable to discharge the parental responsibilities because of mental illness or mental disability, and the condition will continue indefinitely;
- the parent has been convicted of a felony, the nature of which proves parental unfitness or which will result in the absence of the parent for a long period; or
- the best interests of the child argue against the child's remaining in contact with the parents.

When termination is being sought, the court may appoint a guardian *ad litem* for the parent or the child if it believes that it is necessary to protect either's interests. MHPs are sometimes appointed to serve in this role. The court may also order a complete social study and any other evaluation it deems necessary.

What Is the Legal Standard for Termination?

Although the legal standard used in these cases varies by state, the court must evaluate the termination decision in light of the best interests of the child. Several common factors used in making this determination are identifiable. These include

- abandonment of the child if conduct by the parent implies a conscious disregard of the obligations owed by a parent to the child, leading to a destruction of the parent–child relationship;
- parental abuse or neglect if the child has suffered serious physical or emotional harm or sexual abuse by the parent, if there is or has been an ongoing pattern of parental neglect or abuse, if the parents have been unable to provide regular and consistent parenting, or if custody of the child has already been taken away from the parent;
- parental mental illness or disorder if, on the basis of a current evaluation, the parent is unable to discharge parental responsibilities because of the mental illness or disorder, and there is reasonable grounds to believe that the condition will continue for a prolonged indeterminate period;
- parental felony or imprisonment if the parent has been convicted and imprisoned for a felony that proves the unfitness of the parent or if the length of the sentence is such that the child will be deprived of a normal home for a period of years; the former requires consideration of the nature of the act but does not require that the criminal behavior be directed against the child in question; the latter does not indicate automatic termination, rather, there must be an absence of a normal home as a result of the prison sentence; or
- voluntary relinquishment of parental rights if the parents voluntarily relinquished their parental rights to an agency or consented to an adoption.

What Is Involved in the Court Hearing?

The court's primary consideration in these cases is the child's welfare. At the same time, the rights of the parents are to be protected. Both parents are entitled to participate in the hearing, to be represented by counsel, and to show that they are able to raise and care for their child. MHPs often assist the court by assessing parental fitness and the child's best interests. Upon finding that the legal standard for termination has been met, the court orders a termination of parental rights and appoints a guardian for the child. A termination order divests the parent and child of all legal rights, privileges, duties, and obligations with respect to each other except the right of the child to inherit and seek support from the parent. The usual effect of a termination order is to allow the child to be free for adoption. In some states, the court may order postadoptive visitation by the parents or other biological family members.

7

EDUCATION OF CHILDREN

Federal law requires each state to provide education for individuals with disabilities and special needs. In addition, states may require that all children (or just children attending publicly funded schools) be given educational opportunities to meet their unique needs. This broad mandate would include both children with physical, emotional, or mental disabilities as well as children considered gifted because of superior intellect or advanced learning ability. Mental health professionals (MHPs) will be needed to evaluate the special educational needs of children, help design special educational and ancillary services for those children in need, consult with special education personnel, and participate in a program of counseling for the children and parents.

EDUCATION FOR GIFTED AND TALENTED CHILDREN

Gifted and talented children (also known as highly capable students) have been found to have superior intellectual ability, advanced learning ability, or both. Unless special educational services are provided, these children are unlikely to achieve their potential because they will be limited by regular classroom instruction.

How Do Gifted and Talented Children Get Referred for Special Education?

To secure special education services for a gifted and talented child, the child must first be referred for an evaluation to determine his or her need for the services. The referral process is generally less formal than that required for children with disabilities (see the next section). Thus, any person may nominate a highly capable child to receive special education services. Nominations are screened to determine whether the student is likely to meet the eligibility criteria. If the child passes this screening process, he or she will be formally evaluated.

The evaluation process for identifying gifted and talented children is managed by multidisciplinary teams (MDTs), which typically include at least one teacher or other specialist with knowledge in the area of gifted and talented children and an MHP. State law may go further and specify what type of MHP must conduct the evaluation of the child on behalf of the team. One state, for example, allows only certified psychologists and certified school psychologists to evaluate children with special needs. Certified assistant school psychologists or certified psychometrists may administer the evaluation only under the direction of a certified school psychologist.

What Is the Legal Standard to Be Recognized as Gifted and Talented?

To be recognized as a gifted and talented child, the child must meet the state's criteria as determined by the MDT. Such criteria generally include that the child excels in one of the following areas: creative or productive performance, academic aptitude or achievement (e.g., the 95th percentile or above on standardized achievement tests in one or more subject areas), or generalized cognitive ability (e.g., an IQ of 130 or above).

What Must the Evaluation Report Address?

The MDT's written report will typically include

- the reason for the referral;
- educationally relevant medical findings;
- the educational history of the child, including complete documentation of efforts to educate the child in the regular classroom;
- a determination of whether the child's educational problems or needs are related to or resulting from reasons of educational advantage;
- the developmental history of the child;
- the types of tests administered to the child and the results of such tests;

- a recommendation of specific goals and instructional objectives for the child;
- a current vision and hearing screening; and
- an educational evaluation.

What Is the Placement Process for a Gifted and Talented Child?

After being identified as gifted and talented, a student must be provided with educational opportunities that consider his or her unique capabilities and needs. These are organized and monitored through the development of an individualized education plan (IEP). Services may be provided by placement in the school's special education program or alternatively through special programs such as special classes, separate schooling, and supplementary aids and services. The plan must include a statement of the child's present levels of educational performance, the child's annual and short-term instructional goals, the specific services the child will receive, the extent to which the child will be able to participate in regular education, and how the child's progress will be assessed.

Unfortunately, although administrative regulations clearly define how to provide for services and education for children with handicaps (see the section titled Education for Children With Disabilities or Handicaps in this chap.), they usually do not provide clear guidelines for how to meet the needs and abilities of highly gifted students. In general, educational programs are limited by state and local resources.

What Are the Parents' Rights in This Process?

Parents must be given written notice, in their primary language if it is not English, of each step in the special evaluation and placement process. There is usually a requirement that at least one parent consent to the child's evaluation and placement and IEP. Either the parent or the school may initiate an impartial hearing to challenge or show the appropriateness of an action in the process when the other party refuses to proceed with it. If parents request such a hearing, the school must advise them of any free or low-cost legal services. Alternatively, some states have established alternate dispute resolution processes whereby a mediator facilitates an out-of-court settlement of such disagreements. If mediation does not resolve the issue, either party may still request a hearing.

Either party may appeal the hearing officer's decision to the state agency that oversees gifted and talented education (e.g., the Department of Education's Division of Special Education). That agency will then conduct a review of the hearing to determine whether the procedures at the hearing were consistent with legal requirements and that no additional evidence was needed to make an appropriate decision.

EDUCATION FOR CHILDREN WITH
DISABILITIES OR HANDICAPS

Children with handicaps may also be referred to as children with exceptional needs or children with disabilities in state law because of the belief that the term *handicapped* is derogatory. Each state has enacted different laws to provide for these children's education. Some states set age limits (e.g., 3–21 years old) for special education services for these children, and most establish their own criteria for labeling what physical and mental conditions qualify for special services. Some of the conditions include developmental disability, orthopedic impairment, substantial health impairment, learning disability, mental retardation, neurological impairment, multiple handicaps, hearing impairment, communication handicap, visual impairments, and emotional handicap.

What Is the Evaluation Process for a Child With a Disability or Handicap?

To secure special education services for a child with a disability, parents must have the child evaluated to determine his or her need for special educational services. The parents, student, school, or other interested party may initiate the evaluation by making a referral for evaluation to the special education administrator at the child's school or other appropriate personnel (e.g., child study team) in the child's school district. Some states require local school districts to actively conduct programs to identify children with special needs and conditions. When a referral is made, the child's parents must receive written notice of the referral and consent to it. The parent may also obtain a private evaluation conducted by comparable professionals, including MHPs who work outside of the educational system. The appropriate school diagnostic personnel may choose to rely on the outside evaluation in lieu of conducting their own.

The nature of the evaluation that will be conducted depends on the reason for the referral and the type of services sought. State law provides detailed procedures for conducting the assessment. All evaluations are conducted by MDTs that usually include at least one teacher or other specialist with knowledge in the area of the suspected disability(ies), and the evaluations must be conducted in the child's primary language. MHPs are often members of MDTs. If the evaluation is not conducted in English, the evaluator must either be fluent in the child's primary language and in English, use an interpreter, or use test instruments that do not stress spoken language and that are considered valid and reliable performance measures of functioning. The evaluator should also conduct the assessment being conscious of ethnic, cultural, and sexual bias.

Finally, a complete psychological evaluation of the child may be required with one's state specifying who is permitted to perform such an evaluation (e.g., a psychologist or a school psychologist) as well as a comprehensive health evaluation. In some states, the MDT must complete a written report that includes the same factors as those used for gifted and talented children (see the previous section) as well as a determination of whether the child's educational problems or needs are related to or resulting from reasons of educational disadvantage.

What Is the Placement Process for a Child With a Disability or Handicap?

Following the evaluation, a conference must be convened with all relevant personnel, including the school administrative head, the school special education administrator and teacher(s), the child's teacher, the child's evaluators, and one of the child's parents (unless the parent has given written notice that he or she cannot attend). The purpose of the conference is to discuss the results of the evaluation and determine the child's eligibility for special education services. If the child is found to be in need of special education and related services, an IEP will be developed for the child by the special education teacher or by the team and will form the basis by which future progress is measured and adjusted. The IEP must include a statement of the child's present levels of educational performance, the child's annual and short-term instructional goals, the specific services the child will receive, the extent to which the child will be able to participate in regular education, and how the child's progress will be assessed. Some states specify that the IEP must be reviewed and revised at least once each school year and that a complete reevaluation must occur at a minimum of every 3 years. Needed services may be provided to the child by placement in the school's special education program or other special programs (e.g., special classes and separate schooling) and through the use of supplementary aids and services.

What Are the Parents' Rights in This Process?

Parents must be given written notice, in their primary language if it is not English, of each step in the special evaluation and placement process. Parents must also consent to the evaluation, the placement, and to any changes in the placement. Either the parents or the school may initiate a formal challenge to dispute or show the appropriateness of a proposed action if the other refuses to proceed with any part of the process. Some states have established alternative dispute resolution processes whereby a mediator facilitates an out-of-court settlement of such disagreements. If mediation does not resolve the issue, either party may request a hearing.

If parents request such a hearing, the school must advise them of any free or low-cost legal services. A qualified, impartial person who knows the state and federal laws regarding the evaluation, placement, and education of children with handicaps will conduct the hearing. At the hearing, the parties have the right to present evidence and cross-examine witnesses, prohibit the introduction of any evidence that has not been properly disclosed to the other party, present expert witnesses, and be represented by legal counsel and by individuals with special knowledge or training with respect to the problems of children with handicaps. The parents may have additional rights, including the right to examine the child's records, to have the child present, and to open the hearing to the public.

After the hearing is completed, the hearing officer will make a decision on the issue in the case, but the finding may be appealed to the state agency that oversees special education for children with handicaps or disabilities (e.g., the Department of Education's Division of Special Education). That body will then conduct a review of the hearing to determine whether the procedures at the hearing were consistent with the requirements of the law and that no additional evidence was needed to make an appropriate decision.

8

MARRIAGE DISSOLUTION
AND CHILD CUSTODY

Many mental health professionals (MHPs) address therapeutic issues surrounding the breakdown of their clients' interpersonal relationships, yet they are often not aware of or are confused by the complexity of the legal issues in marriage dissolution and child custody cases. Thus, in this chapter, we not only discuss how the law works in this area but also explain how the law may affect an MHP's practice. As a result, an MHP may be able to better understand clients' situations and provide them with accurate information when they are considering or are in the process of terminating a marriage or seeking a change in the custody arrangement for their children.

ANNULMENT

A divorce legally dissolves what was once a valid, functioning marriage; annulment is the process whereby a marriage is declared void and legally never to have existed. This distinction is important for several reasons. Some religions treat marriages that have been annulled differently from those that have been dissolved by divorce. Annulments also have legal significance. An annulled marriage may prevent a deceased person's estate from passing to a surviving ex-spouse under the laws of intestacy (i.e., dying without a will; see chap. 5). Workers' compensation claims may also be affected. For instance, one state's workers' compensation commission contested an annulment because it could result in the state's paying benefits over a longer term. A widowed spouse of a worker receives compensation benefits until the widow remarries; if the second marriage ceases by virtue of an annulment rather than divorce, the widow would be able to reclaim the workers' compensation benefits for the first husband because legally the second marriage never occurred.

Although MHPs are not likely to be involved very often in annulment proceedings, they may be involved in assessing the parties' capacity to consent to marriage (see chap. 5) or in providing therapy to the parties in the annulment process.

What Is the Legal Standard for Annulment?

A marriage may be annulled because it was void from the outset (e.g., incestuous or bigamous) or because it may be voidable for some of the following reasons:

1. A party did not possess the requisite capacity to consent to the marriage. The individual's guardian may petition the court for an annulment in these cases.
2. The consent of either party was obtained by force or duress.
3. One of the parties at the initiation of the marriage intentionally misrepresented or concealed a material fact such that the other person's reason for entering into the marriage is defeated. For example, fraud has been found in cases of concealed pregnancy, pregnancy fathered by a man other than the husband, and concealed drug addiction. In another case, a man represented himself to be a practicing Christian to the woman he was dating but after the marriage stated that he was God. The court concluded that the defendant materially misrepresented himself. However, concealment of mental illness or prior institutionalization has not been found to establish annulment in some cases.
4. Either party was of unsound mind at the time of the marriage.
5. Either party was physically incapable of entering into marriage (e.g., impotence) at the time of the marriage, and such incapacity continues and appears to be incurable.
6. The court finds that annulment would be equitable.

What Is the Outcome of an Annulment?

Although the procedures for obtaining an annulment are generally the same as those for divorce (see the next section), the effect of an annulment is very different. After an annulment, the parties are restored to the status of unmarried persons. In addition, the court may find that because the parties believed in good faith that the marriage was valid, they are given the status of putative spouses (i.e., divorcing spouses), which enables the court to make decisions regarding property division, spousal maintenance, and child custody.

DIVORCE

Marriages are dissolved by annulment, death of one of the partners, or by a judgment of divorce. Prior to 1973, divorce law in most states required one spouse to allege in the divorce petition fault by the other spouse. This changed when most states adopted the Uniform Marriage Act, which allows *no fault* divorces. Instead of having the couple fight over who was at fault for ending the marriage, the court requires the parties to prove that irreconcilable differences led to the marriage being irretrievably broken. The court then concentrates on deciding issues such as property division, child support, spousal maintenance, or child custody (see the next section).

Because many states encourage or mandate mediation to try and avoid divorce or to solve child custody issues, MHPs may contribute to this process by working for court-sponsored or private mediation programs. They may also counsel family members going through and recovering from divorce. Finally, MHPs are often involved in providing assessments relevant to child custody.

What Is the Procedure to Obtain a Divorce?

The first step in dissolving a marriage is for one party to submit a petition to the court alleging that the marriage is irretrievably broken because of irreconcilable differences. The petitioner (the party seeking the divorce) must then have a copy of the petition and a summons to appear in court served on his or her spouse. The spouse then has the opportunity to file a response to the petition before the formal hearing is held.

Refuting an allegation of irreconcilable differences that have caused the marriage to be irretrievably broken is difficult because there may be no legal test in one's state for either irreconcilable differences or an irreparable break in the marriage. If one party denies that the marriage is irretrievably broken by irreconcilable differences, the court must consider all of the relevant factors that may contribute to the possibility that the parties may reconcile and make a factual finding on the issue. Because the burden of maintaining or terminating the marriage is up to the parties and not the court, the court will grant a divorce petition even if only one party steadfastly maintains that the marriage is broken. Alternatively, in some states, the court may grant a divorce if there is proof, in part through testimony given by MHPs, that a party was and is incurably mentally ill or legally insane.

At the time of the filings of the petition and the response, the court may issue a preliminary injunction to either or both spouses prohibiting them from disposing of their property without the written consent of both parties, from disturbing the other spouse or children, and from removing any children then living in that state without the other party's permission. Temporary spousal maintenance or child support may also be granted. Finally, some states encourage or mandate court-operated or private counseling or mediation prior to the court's considering the merits of the divorce petition. The court will then use the counselor's or mediator's report in its decision making.

Fault grounds for divorce still exist in some states. In these states, divorce petitions must state the particular faults that are the basis for the divorce petition. These fault-based grounds include cruel and abusive treatment, desertion or abandonment, conviction of a felony or confinement for a period of time (e.g., 1 year), impotence, and adultery. MHPs may be asked to testify in cases involving allegations of abuse.

What Is the Outcome of a Divorce?

Upon finding that the marriage should be dissolved, the court will make provisions for division of property, support payments, and child custody arrangements. Most states provide for the equitable division of property according to the length of marriage, conduct of the parties, and the respective contributions and needs of the parties. A minority of states are community property states. They divide the couple's community property (all property obtained during the marriage) equally but allow each spouse's separate property (which primarily consists of the property each person brought to the marriage and any gifts or inheritances to the individual) to be retained by that person. For spousal and child support payments, the court may accept a prearranged agreement of the parties or issue an order based on the financial information provided to the court by the parties. To assist the court in making a determination, child support guidelines have been adopted in many states. These are mathematical calculations that determine the amount of child support to be paid. Child custody arrangements are discussed in the following section.

In some states, the divorce decree is final when entered. Unless one of the parties challenges the initial divorce, either spouse may remarry even though the other issues are appealed (e.g., child custody or support payments). However, in other states, the decree is not final until a certain period of time has passed (e.g., 6 months from the date that the petition and summons were served or from the date that the responding spouse appeared in court or after any appeals have been decided).

Some states provide for a shorter version of the divorce procedure previously described. In one state, a summary-disposition procedure is allowed when the parties do not have children, are married for fewer than 5 years, do not have an interest in real property (e.g., real estate), and do not have debt over $4,000 or when their marriage is irretrievably broken because of irreconcilable differences. The parties must sign an agreement about property division and liability allocation and then file a joint petition in court. MHPs may help to influence and facilitate amicable settlements. The court then may dissolve the marriage within 6 months of the filing date.

CHILD CUSTODY AFTER MARITAL DISSOLUTION

Child custody determinations may result from four types of changes in the legal status of a marriage: annulment, legal separation, divorce, and modification of a divorce decree. MHPs are typically involved in the evaluation of the spouses, proposed parent(s), the child, and other relevant persons to provide the court with information on which to base the custody decision in each of these legal actions. These mental status evaluations may culminate in a court appearance as an expert witness.

In some states, one MHP is generally appointed by the court to do the evaluations, with the court maintaining a list of MHPs from which the court may select this evaluator. However, each side may also hire independent MHPs to conduct a separate evaluation and provide testimony. Either side may subpoena MHPs who have provided services to the family, whether diagnostic or therapeutic, to present evidence in court.

Finally, during the divorce proceedings, the court may require both the child and the parents to participate in counseling with an MHP if the dispute is posing a danger to the child's best interests and if counseling would be in the child's best interests. Goals of counseling in these cases include reducing conflict regarding visitation or custody, improving parenting skills, and facilitating communication about the child's best interests.

What Are the Criteria to Establish Court Jurisdiction?

When all relevant parties in a child custody case do not live in the same place, the issue of jurisdiction is raised. State law determines which court may properly make child custody decisions, and the decision usually is based on the domicile of the child and parents. Many states have adopted the Uniform Child Custody Jurisdiction Act, which was enacted to avoid competition among jurisdictions, to ensure that a custody decision is made in the state that can best decide the interests of the child, to deter abductions, and to avoid relitigating cases in different states. Under the act, a state court has jurisdiction in the following instances:

1. The child's home is in the state (a) where the child was recently living (e.g., within 6 months of the start of the custody hearing), even if the child is now absent because of his or her removal by a person claiming custody or for other reasons and (b) where the parent still resides. For instance, if a child and her mother are living in state X at the start of the dissolution proceedings, the court in state X automatically assumes jurisdiction. The physical presence of a child in a state, however, is not sufficient to determine jurisdiction.
2. It is in the best interests of the child that the court assume jurisdiction because
   - the child and at least one parent has significant connections with the state and there is sufficient evidence concerning the child's present or future care, protection, training, and personal relationships in that state;
   - the child is physically present in that state and the child has been abandoned, or it is necessary to protect the child who is neglected, dependent, or abused; or
   - it appears that no other state would have jurisdiction under the above criteria, or another state has declined to exercise jurisdiction because it found that this state is a more appropriate venue to decide the custody of the child.

In this situation, MHPs may be asked to address the nature and quality of the child's relationship with persons in this state as well as the best interests of the child and how that might affect the decision of the court to assume jurisdiction.

What Are the Legal Standards in Custody Determinations?

The court determines custody in accordance with the best interests of the child. This standard takes precedence over individual considerations (e.g., a mother's desire to breastfeed her child). The public policy of many states also favors encouraging both parents to share the rights and responsibilities of raising their child and ensuring that the child receives frequent and continuing contact with both parents after the dissolution, except where such contact is not in the best interests of the child. The court may appoint a guardian *ad litem*, an attorney, or both to represent the child's interests in the proceeding.

In deciding what constitutes the best interests of the child, the court may consider all relevant factors, although some may be specifically set out in the law and therefore are given greater weight. They may include

- the health, safety, and welfare of the child;

- the mental and physical health of all individuals involved;
- the wishes of the parent(s);
- the physical or developmental age of the child and relationship needs with either parent;
- the wishes of the child;
- the interaction and interrelationship of the child with the parent(s), siblings, and any other person who may significantly affect the child's best interests;
- any history that one parent intentionally alienated a child from the other parent (i.e., parental alienation syndrome);
- any history of abuse by one parent against the child or against another parent; the court may require substantial written corroboration of allegations of abuse, including but not limited to written reports by law enforcement agencies, child protective services or other social welfare agencies, courts, and medical facilities or other public agencies or private organizations providing services to victims of sexual abuse or domestic violence;
- the child's adjustment to the home, school, and community; and
- the nature and amount of contact with both parents and which parent is more likely to allow the child frequent and continuing contact with the noncustodial parent.

In addition, the courts in some cases have also considered the acts of adultery by the parent, the age of the child, the gender of the child, and alienation of either parent from the child. In evaluating these factors, the trial court has broad discretion to permit expert testimony (e.g., about attachment and bonding). Some states also provide that unless the court finds that there is no significant risk to the child, no parent shall be given custody or unsupervised visitation with any child if he or she has been convicted of child abuse.

What Are the Potential Custodial Outcomes?

In awarding custody, the court generally follows the following order of preference for custody. First, the court may award custody to both of the child's natural parents jointly or to one of them. Joint custody is an arrangement in which the child lives with each parent on an equal or split-time basis and in which the parents share equally the authority and responsibility for making decisions that significantly affect the welfare of their child. In many states, joint custody is presumed to be in the child's best interests. Second, if neither parent is given custody, the preference goes to the person or persons with whom the child has been living in a wholesome and stable environment (e.g., grandparents). Last, the court may choose any other person or persons who are deemed suitable and able to provide the child with adequate and proper care and guidance. Before the court can grant custody to a nonparent, it usually must find that an award to a parent would be detrimental to the child and that an award to a nonparent is in the child's best interests. Court proceedings considering these issues may be closed to the public.

A parent who is not granted custody of his or her child is entitled to reasonable visitation rights unless the court finds, after a hearing, that visitation would seriously endanger the child's physical, mental, moral, or emotional health. The court may consider the same factors that are used in the custody determination to establish reasonable visitation rights. Some states extend visitation rights to grandparents and siblings in certain circumstances.

What Role Do Mental Status Evaluations Play in Custody Determinations?

As previously discussed, the court may order evaluations and counseling by MHPs in connection with child custody cases. To assist the court in making a custody determination when the parents cannot agree to one, the parties (including the children) may be required to undergo a mental status evaluation in two situations. The law allows a court to order a mental examination whenever the mental condition of a party is at issue.

The court also may order an investigation and report concerning the custodial arrangements for the child. A state may only allow MHPs in designated agencies (e.g., the court's social service agency, the juvenile court, the local probation or welfare department, or a private agency employed by the court) to perform such evaluations. The testimony of MHPs is advisory only; the court is not bound to follow it. Mental status evaluations may also be conducted on a voluntary basis. This usually occurs when one of the parties requests that the MHP conduct an evaluation of the child's parents or proposed parents. If the other party does not wish to participate in the evaluation, the court cannot order the person to do so, although that parental decision may affect the court's ruling.

Although as a general rule, the information obtained by some (e.g., psychologists and psychiatrists) or all MHPs in an examination is privileged (see chap. 3), this is not true for custody evaluations. This information is not privileged because the evaluation is being performed on behalf of the court or because the litigants' mental status is an issue in the case (see chap. 3). In states in which there is no privilege pertaining to all MHPs, MHPs who are not covered in the statute may be subpoenaed to testify regardless of the circumstances of the consultation (see chap. 3).

9

JUVENILE OFFENDERS
BEFORE THE COURT

Children may get into trouble with the law for a variety of reasons ranging from serious criminal activity (e.g., gang violence and murder) to irresponsible conduct (e.g., truancy from school and running away from home). In most states, the juvenile court has the responsibility for hearing complaints about such juveniles. Although the traditional view was to label the juvenile as the problem, some states are involving the family in the court adjudication. These states may refer to complaints against juveniles as a "juvenile–family crisis" or a "family in conflict" and may impose outcomes that involve both the juvenile and the family (e.g., requiring that the family undergo counseling or crisis intervention services).

In this chapter, we discuss the law concerning youth who are brought to juvenile court because they have been found delinquent, dependent, incorrigible, or in need of supervision and services or brought to criminal court because they have been transferred from juvenile court to adult court. Mental health professionals (MHPs) are asked by the courts to evaluate the offending children and the families; provide expert testimony about their mental status, environment, and their amenability to treatment; provide services once treatment is court ordered; serve as members of a crisis intervention unit for the juveniles and their families; and provide counseling to families assigned to a diversion program.

The concepts and terms that one will need to know for this chapter include the following:

- *juveniles* or *minors*—persons who are under the age of 18;
- *dependent children*—those who are (a) in need of proper and effective parental care and control and do not have parents willing to exercise such care and control, (b) abused, or (c) under a certain age and found to have committed an act that would result in adjudication as a delinquent or incorrigible child if committed by an older child;
- *delinquent children*—those who have (a) committed acts that if committed by an adult would be a criminal offense, (b) violated laws specifically addressed to juveniles (e.g., teenage curfew laws), or (c) violated previous orders of the juvenile court;
- *incorrigible children*—those who (a) refuse to obey the reasonable orders of a parent and who are beyond the parent's control, (b) are habitually truant from school, (c) are runaways, (d) habitually injure or endanger the morals or health of themselves or others, (e) violate laws specifically addressed to juveniles (e.g., drinking alcohol), or (f) fail to obey any lawful order of the juvenile court given in a noncriminal action;
- *children in need of services* (CHINS)—a more recent term used in some states for children who would be labeled incorrigible in other states; and
- *persons in need of supervision*—a more recent term used in many states for children who would be labeled incorrigible or CHINS in other states.

JUVENILE COURT AND THE JUSTICE PROCESS

Juvenile courts differ from adult criminal courts in a number of ways. Juvenile courts are considered noncriminal or civil, although the accused individual has the same right to counsel as an adult defendant. Juvenile hearings, unlike criminal trials, generally are not open to the public (unless the child is being tried for murder or is considered a youthful offender in one's state), but the child's parents are expected to be present. Instead of sentencing the minor to prison, the juvenile court can commit the child to the care of the state's department of youth services as well as order the parents to undergo counseling or other services in some states. Finally, with the increasing concern over youth violence, prosecutors are increasingly considering petitioning juvenile courts to transfer cases to criminal court so that juveniles may feel the full brunt of adult criminal laws for their crimes.

How Do Juveniles Get Before the Juvenile Court?

A juvenile enters the juvenile justice system when a law enforcement officer apprehends the child or a complaint is made to the court. The officer may decide to issue a warning to the child and his or her parents instead of taking the child into custody for delinquent actions. If, instead, the officer decides to take the child into custody, the officer may be required to take one of the following steps:

- release the child to his or her parents if they promise to bring the child to court at the proper time,
- bring the child to an officer of the juvenile court,
- take the child to a detention facility pending a hearing before the juvenile court, or
- take the child to a medical facility if the child has a serious condition requiring prompt treatment.

If the juvenile is referred to the juvenile court or to detention, a complaint must be filed immediately with the juvenile court. Complaints may also be filed by any person who writes down specific facts alleging that the child is delinquent, dependent, or in need of supervision and services. For example, school officials may file a petition stating that the child is truant. At that time, the juvenile court will conduct a preliminary investigation and hearing. Often, juvenile probation officers conduct these investigations to determine whether the facts, if true, are sufficient to bring the child within the court's jurisdiction and whether they appear serious enough without further investigation to warrant some form of court action. This may include referral for an MHP evaluation. Alternatively, all complaints and referrals may be screened through a court intake service.

Once screened, cases may be dismissed, diverted, or referred for court action. Pretrial diversion agreements and programs are common and usually involve the agreement of the juvenile or his or her family to certain conditions (e.g., community service, restitution, counseling, or a fine) instead of prosecution.

What Happens at Juvenile Court Hearings?

If court action is warranted, a formal hearing is scheduled, and the child is released to await the hearing, unless

- the child is likely to leave the area,
- the parents are likely to remove the child from the area,
- the parents or guardian are not giving the child adequate care and protection,
- the child has no parents or guardian,
- the child is dangerous to him- or herself,

- the child may threaten the safety of the community, or
- the child has a history of delinquency and crime and is likely to commit an offense if released.

After setting a time for a hearing and giving notice to the child and his or her parents, guardian, or custodian (hereinafter parents), any witnesses needed for the hearing will be served with subpoenas. The court may divide the hearings into a number of stages (advisory, detention, adjudication, and disposition) or handle all matters at one time. If the court finds that the facts alleged in the petition are true, the child will be placed under the jurisdiction of the court.

At the advisory hearing, the court will advise the child and parents of their rights to counsel, to remain silent through any and all phases of the hearing, and to call witnesses on the child's behalf. If the child or parents request counsel, the court will recess the hearing and order that counsel be appointed for the parties. If the child does not have parents or a guardian, the court will likely appoint a guardian *ad litem* who will represent the child's interests. The court may then set a time for the adjudication hearing.

At the detention hearing, the court will hear reasons by the petitioner or probation officer as to why the child should be detained or continue to be detained. A court may detain the child if it has reason to believe that the child committed the acts alleged in the petition and if one of the previously listed criteria is again met. The detention hearing may be held without the presence of the child's parents if they cannot be found or fail to appear. Some states require that detention hearings occur every 2 weeks prior to the disposition hearing to ensure that the juvenile is being justly detained.

At the adjudication hearing, the court decides the issue of delinquency or need for supervision and services. After the state proves and the court finds that the child committed the alleged delinquent offense, a disposition hearing is held. At the *disposition hearing*, the court decides what will happen to the child who has been found to be delinquent or in need of services and supervision. The disposition depends on the classification and particular needs of the child (e.g., services for a mental, emotional, or personality disorder or a developmental disability). Generally, the juvenile probation officer or MHPs will make such investigations as the court directs and submit a written report and recommendations to the court before the hearing takes place. The court may also order physical, psychiatric, and psychological examinations of the child. A parent who wishes to provide the court with the testimony of a privately retained mental health professional who conducted an independent examination would be able to do so.

What Are Possible Juvenile Court Outcomes?

The court may place the child with a wide variety of people or institutions as the final disposition. Many of the placements are made subject to supervision by the probation department or Child Protective Services. Placements may include

- the care of the parents, subject to supervision;
- a probation department, subject to such conditions that the court may impose;
- a reputable citizen of good moral character, subject to supervision;
- a private agency or institution, subject to supervision;
- a suitable school;
- a supervised independent-living program;
- the department of corrections without further directions as to placement by the department; or
- a maternal or paternal relative, subject to supervision.

The court may also order treatment by MHPs as well as medical and educational services as part of the child's rehabilitation program. Some placements (e.g., to a state's department of youth services) may require and provide mental health services to the child. If the court awards custody of the child to the state's department of corrections or to an institution or agency, it must transmit all mental health reports to it. In addition, the court may order the child to make full or partial restitution (i.e., financial compensation) to the victim of an offense and assess a reasonable fine if it determines that it will aid rehabilitation. Such an assessment must take into account the nature of the offense and child-specific factors (e.g., mental condition and earning capacity).

Finally, in considering an appropriate disposition for a juvenile, the court will consider all of the alternative dispositions available to it, including, as previously noted, probation, foster care, and placement in a public or private institution. It must consider where a minor would benefit from placement and if he or she poses a danger to the community given any violent propensities (e.g., causing damage or stealing property). Courts will also take into account the child's mental illness or developmental disability in reaching its decision.

COMPETENCY OF JUVENILES TO STAND TRIAL

Minors who appear before the juvenile court have most of the constitutional and procedural protections that are available to adult criminal defendants, including the right against self-incrimination and the right to be aware of and participate in any proceedings against them. However, some protections may not be as strong for juveniles as for adults because of the state's interest in protecting children. For example, the child may not have the right to a jury trial.

Some states' law provides that juveniles must meet the same standards to stand trial that adult criminal defendants do (see chap. 9). To be considered competent to stand trial, the juvenile must be able to understand the nature of the charges against him or her and the nature of the proceedings and be able to assist in his or her defense. The court may order an MHP's examination for competency to stand trial if the judge has reason to suspect there is a problem. Although ironic, this process could be applied to children solely because of their "tender years" and immaturity. If found incompetent to stand trial, the child is not subject to further proceedings in juvenile court until made competent, but the court may order commitment for mental health services.

In states whose law does not specifically address the issue of juvenile competence to stand trial, the juvenile's mental status is presumed to be part of the information that the court will consider in fashioning a disposition.

NONRESPONSIBILITY DEFENSE IN JUVENILE PROCEEDINGS

In some states, children under a certain age (e.g., 14 years old) are considered incapable of committing crimes as a matter of law. In states in which the child is considered capable of committing a crime or delinquent act, he or she may, depending on the state, have the right to raise the insanity defense as a defense to the allegation. The legal standard for such a defense is typically the same for juveniles as for adults in that jurisdiction (see chap. 13). The court may order an examination by MHPs to help in making a disposition in the case.

Proof of insanity does not limit the ability of the juvenile court to make a finding of delinquency in some states, even though the insanity defense would be a complete defense in adult court. Other states require that delinquency proceedings be dismissed if there is a finding of legal insanity. Generally, a finding of insanity results in the court's ordering rehabilitative measures such as psychotherapy or commitment to mental health or mental retardation services. State law may limit the length of commitment (e.g., no longer than to age 18 or 21).

TRANSFER OF JUVENILES TO STAND TRIAL AS ADULTS

Historically, minors were tried in the juvenile court for their misdeeds and crimes. Even today, children under a certain legal age who are charged with the worst of crimes (e.g., murder) will be prosecuted in juvenile court as a delinquency matter. Yet states are increasingly under pressure to treat minors as adults when they commit particularly serious crimes. For this reason, some states have given the juvenile courts authority to sentence a new category of offender (e.g., youthful offenders) to adult or juvenile penalties for committing an offense involving the infliction of or threat of serious bodily harm or in which a gun was used. Other states have considered the total elimination of the juvenile court because of a shift in public attitudes toward getting tough on juvenile crime.

But perhaps the most commonly discussed practice today is the trend in many states to transfer minors to the criminal courts. MHPs may contribute to the transfer hearing on behalf of the court, the prosecuting attorney, or the defense attorney. In performing this role, the MHP will likely conduct an assessment of the minor and be asked to make predictive evaluations of how the juvenile would fare in the juvenile justice system as compared with the adult penal system. If the court transfers the case to adult court, the child is treated as an adult in most ways (i.e., the child will generally be protected from contact with adult prisoners).

A request for a transfer hearing may be made by any of the parties, although the prosecutor usually requests it. After the request is made, an investigation is conducted and a report is made available to all the parties before the hearing. The report must contain the results of an evaluation of the child, including social background, previous delinquent history, all social records that are to be made available to the court at the transfer hearing, and any other relevant information gathered.

During the hearing, the court must determine that an offense has been committed, that probable cause exists to believe that the juvenile committed the crime, and that there are reasonable grounds to believe that the child meets the criteria for transfer to adult court.

The criteria for transfer to adult court typically include

- whether the child is at least a certain age (e.g., 16 years old);
- whether the child has a history of contacts with the juvenile court and further treatment is not likely to be beneficial;
- whether the crime is so serious that the child will be incarcerated beyond age 18;
- the seriousness of the alleged offense to the community and whether protection of the community requires transfer to adult court;
- whether the alleged offense was committed in an aggressive, violent, premeditated, or willful manner;
- whether the alleged offense was against persons or against property, with greater weight being given to offenses against persons, especially if personal injury resulted;
- the desirability of trial and disposition of the entire offense in one court in which the juvenile's associates in the alleged offense are adults;
- the sophistication and maturity of the juvenile as determined by consideration of the home, environmental situation, emotional attitude, and pattern of living;

- the record and previous history of the juvenile; and
- the prospect for adequate protection of the public and the likelihood of reasonable rehabilitation of the juvenile (if found to have committed the alleged offense) by use of the procedures, services, and facilities currently available to the juvenile court.

10

STATE INTERVENTIONS AND SERVICES FOR INDIVIDUALS WITH SPECIAL NEEDS

The states provide services for individuals with special needs, including people with mental illness, alcohol and substance abuse issues, and developmental disabilities (e.g., mental retardation). This category also includes individuals who receive treatment and care because they have been victims of domestic violence, are released after serving a sentence for a sexual offense, or are dying. Mental health professionals (MHPs) are involved in the assessment and treatment of these individuals and in testifying in court.

PEOPLE WITH MENTAL ILLNESS

State law provides for the care of people with mental illness in a number of ways. Some people may be eligible to receive inpatient or outpatient mental health services through their private heath care plans or plans funded by the state or federal governments (e.g., state health plans for indigent people and Medicaid). State law also provides for voluntary civil admission and involuntary civil commitment of persons with mental illness to state-operated inpatient facilities or to outpatient services (labeled *assertive community treatment* in some states). MHPs are involved in the admission and commitment process in evaluating the person, testifying in court as to their findings, and providing services. In this chapter, we discuss these two types of mental health treatment.

What Is the Difference Between Voluntary Admission and Involuntary Commitment?

There are differences between voluntary and involuntary hospitalization. Generally, voluntary admission is permissible for those people with a variety of mental, emotional, or personality disorders, whereas involuntary commitment is only authorized for those people who meet a set of more restrictive standards listed in state law (see the section titled What Is Involved in the Involuntary Commitment of People With Mental Illness? in this chap.). Many states have an explicit policy favoring voluntary treatment over involuntary commitment because the latter type of commitment may generate substantial costs to the state and involves a loss of liberty to the person being committed.

What Is Involved in Voluntary Admission?

Voluntary admission may be requested by

- any person 18 years of age or older;
- a guardian who has authority to seek admission for his or her ward (see chaps. 5 and 6);
- the parent(s) of a minor under the age of 18, although at least one state limits parental admission to minors under the age of 16; or
- a minor who meets a state's age limit (e.g., at least 16 years old).

The medical director of the proposed admitting facility or the admitting MHP must believe that the person needs evaluation or will benefit from treatment for a mental, emotional, or personality disorder for that person to be admitted. These conditions that qualify for voluntary treatment are generally broader than those allowed for involuntary commitment (see the next section). For example, in one state, involuntary commitment is limited to persons with a mental disorder, which is defined to exclude drug addiction, alcoholism, and personality disorders. However, these conditions may be treated if the person is voluntarily admitted to a treatment facility.

If the person has recovered or if he or she is no longer benefiting from treatment, he or she will typically be released promptly. Voluntary admission, however, does not mean that a person will be discharged immediately on request. If the facility finds that the person meets the criteria for involuntary commitment, then it will file a petition for court-ordered treatment and typically be allowed to hold the person for 72 hours for the court to act on the petition. Thus, the person's right to leave the facility is not absolute, even though the original admission was voluntary.

Just prior to admission, the person or the parent or guardian must sign an informed consent form. This form should not only discuss treatment issues (see chap. 2) but also cover any confidentiality and privilege communication limitations, the fact that the voluntary evaluation may result in a petition for involuntary treatment or for guardianship in the case of an adult patient (see chap. 5), and a list of the rights that the person is afforded by the institution. Some of these rights will be required by state law.

What Is Involved in the Involuntary Commitment of People With Mental Illness?

Most state laws provide for two routes that may be used to involuntarily commit a person. The first route generally consists of a petition for a court-ordered commitment, a court review of the petition, an order for commitment, and an appeals process. Some states also mandate a series of steps before the petition may be filed, such as requiring an application for a court-ordered evaluation and an evaluation or screening before the petition is filed. The second route, emergency commitment, authorizes a police officer to take a person into custody if the officer believes that the person is likely to suffer or inflict serious bodily harm without immediate hospitalization and transport the person to an appropriate facility. Because involuntary commitment involves a significant restriction of a person's liberty and because of past abuses of the commitment process, there are many legally mandated procedures that must be followed to ensure that the person's rights are protected. In addition, the person has the right to appeal a commitment decision by the court.

What Is the Legal Standard for Involuntary Commitment?

All states allow for the involuntary commitment of persons with mental illness if they are a danger to others, a danger to self, or gravely disabled. Some states have added a fourth standard that allows for commitment if the person is in need of supervision, care, and treatment and no less restrictive alternative is appropriate. These criteria will be applied to both adults and juveniles who are petitioned for involuntary commitment.

What Does a Screening Process Involve?

Some states begin the long-term commitment process by requiring a screening and an evaluation of the proposed patient. In these states, any person may apply for a screening of another individual. The person generally should include the following information in his or her application:

- biographical information concerning the proposed patient;
- dates and places of the proposed patient's previous hospitalization, if any;
- a statement that the proposed patient is believed to meet the state's criteria for commitment and why the person believes this to be true;
- a statement as to why less restrictive alternatives are inappropriate; and
- information about the relationship of the applicant to the proposed patient.

Within a certain period of time (e.g., 48 hours) of the receipt of the application, the agency, or designated MHP in some states, in charge of screening the proposed patient may have some of the following duties and responsibilities:

- to review the application and investigate the facts alleged in the petition;
- to interview the applicant;
- to interview the proposed patient;
- to explain the application procedures; and
- to attempt to persuade the proposed patient to receive an evaluation or other services on a voluntary basis, when appropriate.

If the proposed patient accompanies the applicant to the screening agency, the screening evaluation will be conducted at that time. If the proposed patient does not go with the applicant, the screening may be conducted at his or her home or wherever he or she can be found. Note, however, that the proposed patient cannot be detained or forced to undergo the evaluation against his or her will unless the person meets the criteria for emergency admission (see the section titled What Is Involved in the Emergency Commitment of People With Mental Illness? in this chap.). In some states, the agency does not need to interview the proposed patient. An investigation of the facts in the application and an interview with the applicant may provide a sufficient foundation for a commitment petition. In other states, a personal interview is mandatory.

After the screening evaluation has been completed, the agency or designated MHP prepares a report of opinions and conclusions. If the report concludes that there is reasonable cause to believe that that person meets the legal standard for the specified type of commitment, the screening agency or designated MHP also files a petition for a court-ordered evaluation. This prepetition screening process results in allowing only the agency or MHP to file a petition in court for a court-ordered evaluation.

The agency may also be required to contact the county attorney if it finds that the proposed patient presents a danger to others. The county attorney may then recommend that a criminal investigation be conducted if warranted, that the agency file the petition, or that no further proceedings be conducted. This recommendation is included with the petition filed at the court.

On receiving a petition for evaluation from the agency, the court will determine whether the person will undergo the evaluation on an inpatient or outpatient basis. If the person is already involuntarily hospitalized, the court will appoint an attorney to represent the person during this process if one is needed. The proposed patient may be taken into custody and required to submit to an inpatient evaluation if (a) the court finds reasonable cause to believe that the proposed patient is likely to present a danger to self or others before the hearing on the court-ordered treatment or (b) the person fails to appear at a scheduled outpatient evaluation. The evaluation must take place within a certain period (e.g., 72 hours or 4 days) after the court approves the evaluation. A clinical record with details of all medical and mental health services received by the person during the evaluation must be kept.

If it is determined that further evaluation is not appropriate, the person will be released. If it is determined that the person meets the state's criteria for involuntary commitment, then the evaluation agency or MHP will prepare, sign, and file a petition for court-ordered treatment (see the next section). If no petition is filed, the person must be released at the end of the evaluation period.

What Is the Commitment Process Like Without a Screening Process?

Any person may file an involuntary commitment petition with the court. The commitment petition for such court-ordered treatment may be required to include

- facts that show that the person meets the legal standard for commitment;
- a claim that there is no less restrictive alternative for this person other than hospitalization;
- a statement that the patient is unwilling to accept treatment or incapable of accepting it voluntarily; and
- affidavits of witnesses, physicians, and/or MHPs that describe the behavior of the person supporting the need for commitment.

State law requires that a hearing on the petition be held within a certain period of time (e.g., 14 days of the filing) and that the proposed patient receive notice of the hearing. Prior to the hearing, the person has the right to be evaluated by an independent MHP. If the person is unable to afford it, the court is required to appoint an independent evaluator acceptable to the patient from a list of MHPs who are willing to serve in this capacity. The patient also may have the right to

- be free of the influences or effects of drugs, medications, or other treatment that hampers preparing for or participating in the hearing;
- review and copy records;
- have an attorney;
- present evidence;
- subpoena and cross-examine witnesses;
- cross-examine opposing witnesses;
- have the hearing in camera (i.e., private); and
- obtain a certified transcript of the hearing.

In most states, the person filing the commitment petition (the petitioner) must show proof by clear and convincing evidence that the proposed patient meets the standard for involuntary commitment. As part of this showing, the petitioner may be required to present the testimony of two witnesses acquainted with the patient at the time of the alleged mental disorder and the testimony of two physicians or MHPs who evaluated the patient.

What Are the Potential Outcomes of the Commitment Hearing?

If the petitioner has not proven the case, the court will dismiss the petition and discharge the patient. If the case is substantiated, the court will order commitment of the proposed patient. Its order will consist of outpatient treatment or inpatient treatment in a mental health treatment agency, a Veteran's Administration hospital, state hospital, or private hospital. Each state sets different time limits on commitments (e.g., a maximum of 6 months), and these may be related to the reason for commitment (e.g., danger to self, 90 days; danger to others, 180 days; and gravely disabled, 365 days). The court may require a written treatment plan from the facility that the person is being committed to. Finally, if the person is found to be incompetent to consent to or refuse services (e.g., psychotropic medication), the court will order an investigation into that matter. If the investigation confirms such need, the court will appoint a guardian *ad litem* for the person.

What Is Involved in the Release or Less Restrictive Alternative Treatment of People With Mental Illness?

The patient must be discharged at the expiration of the period of treatment ordered unless the person accepts voluntary treatment or a new petition is filed. A patient may be released from treatment prior to the expiration of the court-ordered period when, in the opinion of the medical director of the agency, the patient no longer meets the criteria for commitment. The medical director may be obligated to first give notice to the court, any victim or relative of the patient, and any person found by the court to have a legitimate reason for receiving such notice. The purpose of such notice is to allow those persons to request that the court hold an evidentiary hearing to determine whether the patient should be released.

In some states, a patient who was originally committed to an inpatient facility may obtain a conditional outpatient release if, after consultation with the staff, the medical director determines that the patient

- no longer requires continuous inpatient hospitalization,
- will be more appropriately treated with an outpatient treatment plan,
- will follow a prescribed outpatient treatment plan, and
- will not likely become dangerous or suffer more serious physical harm or serious illness if he or she follows a prescribed outpatient treatment plan.

The medical director of the inpatient commitment facility must issue a written outpatient treatment plan, which will include the patient's medication, supervision, living requirements, and the entity authorized to supervise the plan. The outpatient treatment may only last as long as the time left in the original court commitment order. The notice requirements previously described may also apply if the patient was committed because he or she was a danger to others. The medical director may rescind or modify an order for conditional outpatient treatment if the patient fails to comply with the terms of the treatment plan or if outpatient treatment is no longer appropriate.

What Is Involved in the Emergency Commitment of People With Mental Illness?

Any person may make a written application to the court for the emergency admission of another. The danger presented by the proposed patient must be sufficiently compelling to justify bypassing the regular admission procedures previously described (e.g., imminent and serious danger to self or others). If the presented reasons are sufficient, the judge may issue a warrant to bring the person to court or to a mental health facility to be evaluated. If the court finds that the person creates a likelihood of serious harm if not hospitalized, the court may order an emergency commitment for a limited period of time (e.g., 10 days), during which a petition for a regular commitment hearing may be developed.

A qualified member of a mental health agency also may sign an application for emergency admission to a qualified mental health facility. The application describes the reasons for believing that failure to hospitalize would lead to serious harm as a result of the person's mental disorder.

Finally, in some states, a person in the presence of a police officer or the police officer him- or herself may make a telephone application to an agency. After determining that reasonable cause exists to support an emergency examination, the admitting MHP of the evaluation agency may advise the police officer to take the person into custody and to transport him or her to the facility. If the officer is unable to use the telephone and has probable cause to believe the person meets the criteria for emergency commitment, the officer may transport the person to an agency without specific authorization to do so.

Upon presentation of the person for emergency admission, an admitting officer of the mental health agency must determine whether the person meets the criteria for emergency commitment. If the person does not meet the criteria, the agency must release the person. If the person meets the criteria, the agency will admit the person for a short period of time (e.g., 2–3 days). The proposed patient may be released sooner if the director of the facility or another authorized person (e.g., the attending MHP) determines that it is appropriate.

A person undergoing an emergency commitment typically has the right to

- be offered treatment;
- refuse treatment; however, seclusion or mechanical or pharmacological restraints may be used as emergency measures for the safety of the person or others;
- have his or her guardian, or if none, a member of the family (other than the person who has made application for emergency admission) be given notice of the person's presence at the agency;
- have the facility director inquire into the need to safeguard and preserve the person's personal property or premises; and
- be advised of his or her right to consult an attorney and the right to an appointed attorney if the person cannot afford one.

What Are a Person's Rights During Commitment?

The person has numerous rights during commitment. Some of the more important ones are

- the right to examine the written treatment program and the medical record unless the attending physician determines that such an examination is clinically contraindicated;
- the right to consult with counsel (e.g., at least once every 60 days) while undergoing court-ordered treatment;

- the right to judicial review at certain time intervals (e.g., every 60 days) at which time the court may review the additional material presented and enter its order without necessity of further hearing;
- the right to make personal, confidential phone calls and to have visitors, subject to reasonable limitations as the individual in charge of the agency may direct;
- the right to be free from excessive or unnecessary medication;
- the right not to be subjected to certain procedures (e.g., experimental research, shock treatment, psychosurgery, lobotomy, other types of brain surgery, or sterilization) without the person's or guardian's informed consent, consultation with an attorney, or a court order authorizing the procedure; and
- the right to be advised of these rights, both orally and in writing.

Two additional rights often talked about are the right to treatment and the right to refuse treatment. When people voluntarily contract with an MHP to receive services, they have the right to receive the services that they pay for. Conversely, competent adults have the right to refuse treatment that they voluntarily sought. The situation is more complex in involuntary imposed services. There is no right to treatment during involuntary commitment, although states would find it difficult to justify continued commitment if no attempts at treatment were made. The treatment, however, can be psychotropic medication without any psychosocial intervention. In some states, involuntarily committed persons have the right to refuse treatment except in emergency circumstances. If they refuse the treatment, they then cannot argue that they should be released because they are not receiving treatment.

Competent adults may designate a health care proxy who is authorized to make treatment or nontreatment decisions in the event that the person becomes incompetent. They can accomplish this through executing a power of attorney or an advanced directive instrument limited to mental health care.

For persons seeking voluntary treatment who are believed to be incompetent to consent to treatment (see chap. 2), a court will render a judgment about the individual's competency (see chap. 5). If a person is found to be incompetent, the court will appoint either a guardian (i.e., substitute decision maker) or a guardian *ad litem* (guardian over a specific issue, such as making treatment decisions). For involuntary treatment, the person typically is not required to consent to services, but the person would have to be competent to ask for or implement his or her rights. If an MHP had any reason to assume that the person who was involuntarily committed lacked the competency to make personal decisions, the staff, in most states, would petition the court for a judgment.

Are Mental Health Professionals Liable for Working With People With Mental Illness?

MHPs who have acted in good faith pursuant to the law are likely to be legally immune from civil and criminal liability for evaluating and testifying about individuals who are the subject of a commitment petition.

PEOPLE WITH ALCOHOLISM

State law provides for voluntary treatment and involuntary commitment of those persons who are seriously disabled by alcoholism. Rather than criminalizing and jailing untreated persons with alcoholism, laws in some states were changed to provide them with a continuum of care with the focus of the legal intervention being treatment. Some states have also passed laws that require state agencies to provide educational services regarding the causes, effects, and treatment of intoxication and alcoholism. MHPs may be part of a multidisciplinary evaluation and treatment team under these laws and provide services in a variety of settings.

How Does a Person Obtain Voluntary Alcoholism Treatment?

A person who is intoxicated may apply for emergency alcoholism treatment at a local alcoholism reception center. Any person with alcoholism (even if not intoxicated), as defined by state law, may also apply for evaluation and treatment directly to any treatment facility. In most states, if the applicant is a minor or an incompetent person, either the parent or legal guardian must make the application. Other states allow some minors to voluntarily consent to treatment (e.g., age 16 years or older). If a person is refused admission at a private facility for financial reasons, the administrator may be legally obligated to refer the person to a public facility, if appropriate.

A person with alcoholism who is brought before the court and charged with a crime may undergo evaluation and treatment if both the court and the person agree. The period of treatment may have a time limit (e.g., not to exceed 30 days). During that time, the criminal proceedings are suspended.

How Do People Obtain Emergency Alcoholism Treatment?

Any individual may bring a person who is intoxicated to a local alcoholism reception center for an emergency evaluation and treatment if the person threatened or attempted to inflict physical harm on him- or herself or another, is likely to inflict future harm on him- or herself or another unless admitted, or is incapacitated by alcohol. Further, a police officer who has reasonable cause to believe that a person is intoxicated in a public place and is a danger to him- or herself or others may use reasonable force to transport the person to a local alcoholism reception center. Police officers may remain at the facility to provide adequate security and protection. If there is no local center or other approved facility or if the local center is filled to capacity, then the officer may transport the person to a detention facility.

Discharge From Services Provided on an Emergency Basis

The law may specify how long a person may be kept on an emergency basis at a detention facility or local alcoholism reception center. In some states, any person taken to a detention facility must be released when the person is no longer intoxicated, after a certain time period (e.g., 12 hours), or at any time to a responsible person. Persons taken to a local alcoholism reception center must be released within a certain time period (e.g., no more than 24 hours) after the person requests discharge or when the center administrator determines that the grounds for admission no longer exist. Some states allow a person to be involuntarily detained for up to 48 hours.

How Do People Receive Involuntary Alcoholism Treatment and Commitment?

Typically, a police officer, relative, guardian, physician, or administrator of a local alcoholism center may file a petition for involuntary commitment with the appropriate court in the county where the person lives or where the center is located. The petition usually must allege that the person has alcoholism and has not substantially benefited from previous treatment and that there is a reasonable risk of serious harm or illness in the near future if the person does not receive treatment.

The court must schedule an immediate hearing (e.g., within 5 days) of the filing of the petition. The person may have to be evaluated by a physician and/or an MHP. At the hearing, the person may have the right to

- be provided with counsel if the person is unable to afford one,
- be represented by counsel at every stage of the proceeding,
- be present at the hearing,
- present evidence and witnesses,
- cross-examine opposing witnesses, and
- request that the hearing be transcribed.

The hearing is generally conducted in an informal manner. If the court finds that the person meets the criteria for involuntary commitment, the court must order commitment to a treatment facility for a certain period of time (e.g., not to exceed 90 days). For longer commitments, the court may also order that the receiving treatment facility develop a treatment plan for the person soon after admission. The treatment plan is based on a comprehensive assessment of the person's physical, mental, and social functioning, including the person's primary problems and treatment objectives, methods, and costs. One state, for example, requires an HIV/AIDS risk intervention with each client.

Discharge From Services Following Involuntary Alcoholism Treatment and Commitment

A person committed under such laws may be discharged before the end of the treatment period if the administrator of the treatment facility determines that the person is no longer incapacitated by alcohol, treatment in the facility is no longer adequate or appropriate for the person's needs, or further treatment is unlikely to bring about significant improvement in the person's condition. For example, some states provide for a conditional release to a less restrictive treatment program (e.g., a residential inpatient treatment program, transitional living arrangement, or a work training program), when it is deemed appropriate. Involuntary commitment, however, will automatically terminate at the expiration of the court order. The facility may then file a petition for recommitment using the same legal standards applied to the original commitment. However, there may be a limit to the number of times a person may be recommitted. In the alternative, treatment may continue beyond the automatic discharge if it is appropriate and the person agrees.

At the conclusion of the involuntary treatment, state law may require that the facility evaluate the person's progress, propose an aftercare treatment plan, and assist the person in finding a voluntary reentry program in the person's community. The facility may also be required to monitor the person's condition for a period of time after discharge (e.g., at least 6 months), including the person's use of the local alcoholism reception center's services.

PEOPLE WITH SUBSTANCE ABUSE PROBLEMS

Some states provide for voluntary treatment and involuntary commitment of persons with major substance abuse problems (i.e., persons with drug dependence or addiction). The procedure is often the same as that described for people with alcoholism (see the previous section). In addition to these more traditional methods of referring persons with substance abuse problems to treatment, a new legal procedure, drug treatment court, is used in some states for cases involving the possession or purchasing of drugs or of other nonfelony drug-related charges. MHPs may provide evaluative and therapeutic services and testify in court in both types of cases.

What Are Drug Courts?

After the "drug war" in the late 1980s resulted in a dramatic increase in drug-related prosecutions, courts started to implement new procedures with which to handle cases involving drug offenders. Two general models for processing drug offense cases have emerged: the expedited drug case method (EDCM) and the drug treatment court (DTC).

Courts using the EDCM rely on the traditional techniques of criminal case processing, including the adversarial relationship (i.e., prosecution vs. defense attorney); judge as detached arbiter; and punishment, probation or parole, and community supervision as consequences for convicted drug offenders. The EDCM does not emphasize treatment and recovery. It concentrates on speeding up the judicial process to eliminate or deal with the increase in drug cases. The EDCM also facilitates the early resolution of cases by providing clear guidelines for plea offers; using defendant waivers to bypass the grand jury process; and setting advanced dates for plea negotiations, trials, and motions.

A DTC addresses the drug addiction behind the person's offenses. A DTC can be defined as a cooperative system in which local law enforcement, community drug treatment facilities, and courts work together to instigate and supervise the treatment of certain categories of drug offenders. By giving drug offenders the opportunity to overcome their addiction and correct their addictive behaviors, DTCs aim to reduce reoffending and docket loads. Rather than seeing drug addiction as solely a criminal behavior, DTCs believe that substance abuse is a chronic, progressive, relapsing biopsychosocial disease that can be successfully treated. A biopsychosocial approach addresses the biological, psychological, and social factors that are interwoven into how a person developed and maintains his or her addiction.

The methods and means of DTCs vary according to the needs, problems, and resources of the local community. Although the structure of DTCs varies by state and local jurisdictions, they have a common goal—drug treatment instead of incarceration or probation for addicted offenders. Thus, some common elements of DTCs include

- immediate intervention;
- a nonadversarial adjudication process;
- a hands-on judicial approach to the defendant's or participant's treatment program;
- clearly defined rules and structured goals in the participant's treatment program; and
- a DTC team (judge, prosecutor, defense counsel, treatment provider, and corrections personnel) approach.

The planning and funding of drug courts is supported by legislation in a number of states, the Office of Drug Court Programs in the Department of Justice, and Title V of the Violent Crime Control and Law Enforcement Act of 1994, which specifically allocated federal finds for drug court support.

Who May Participate in Drug Treatment Courts and When Do They Start Treatment?

Originally, DTCs did not attempt to treat people with all types of addiction (e.g., people with alcoholism). Initially, DTCs concentrated on cases involving illicit drug use by adults. However, "second-generation" DTCs are expanding their efforts. Some DTCs provide programs directed specifically at persons with alcoholism. Others have created juvenile and family DTCs to address the substance abuse problems of juveniles and other family members.

Despite this trend of expanding access, DTCs still generally deal with adult drug cases on the basis of certain court or legislatively prescribed criteria. The criteria for admission to a DTC program vary from court to court, but most courts focus on the individual's inability to stop abusing or using illegal drugs without the criminal justice system's involvement. Thus, eligibility criteria generally consider two issues: (a) the extent of a potential participant's drug involvement and (b) the relative risk that a potential participant would pose to public safety.

Defendants typically become involved with DTCs through two different routes: preadjudication (diversion or deferred prosecution) and postadjudication (deferred sentencing or entry of judgment). The preadjudication DTC approach generally occurs shortly after being charged when a defendant waives his or her right to a speedy trial and enters a treatment program. If he or she fails to complete the program, his or her charges are reinstated and brought to trial (adjudicated). The postadjudicative approach involves trying the case and finding the offender guilty or requiring a guilty plea. However, the defendant's sentence and incarceration are deferred until either he or she successfully completes the treatment program or the court terminates the treatment program for lack of progress.

What Interventions Are Used by the Drug Treatment Court?

The DTC relies on treatment programs that are designed to teach participants skills necessary to cope with and overcome their addiction. Treatment methods generally include group, individual, and/or family therapy; weekly, random urinalysis testing; and attendance at scheduled DTC hearings. Outpatient or inpatient counseling together with regular drug testing is the most widely used DTC treatment program. A participant may be assigned to residential treatment if he or she cannot maintain a drug-free lifestyle without constant supervision. In addition, all DTCs follow the 12-step recovery process of Alcoholics Anonymous and Narcotics Anonymous and encourage participants to attend regular meetings. Finally, other therapeutic approaches are used in various jurisdictions (e.g., acupuncture).

In most drug courts, treatment is designed to last at least 1 year. However, the length of time a person spends in a treatment program depends on his or her compliance with treatment protocol. Many DTCs use incentives and sanctions that increase or decrease the duration of an individual's treatment program to encourage adherence to treatment and court rules. Because relapse is expected, DTCs generally have criteria that allow courts to "recycle" individuals through a particular treatment phase during a relapse, instead of terminating them from treatment. Thus, this procedure may extend the length of time a person remains in the treatment program. For this reason and because the length of programs normally exceeds the potential jail time for a drug possession offense, some defense attorneys and other concerned groups (e.g., civil libertarians) have expressed concerns about these programs.

PEOPLE WITH DEVELOPMENTAL DISABILITIES

Although the definition of developmental disability varies by state, it generally refers to a severe and chronic disability caused by mental retardation, cerebral palsy, epilepsy, autism, or other neurological disorder like mental retardation. Usually the disability must have begun before the person turned 18 and resulted in (a) a substantial limitation in the person's functioning (self-care, receptive and expressive language, learning, mobility, self-direction, capacity for independent living, and economic self-sufficiency) and (b) a need for extended interdisciplinary care of a unique nature. Some persons with developmental disabilities are also visually or auditorily handicapped.

The law recognizes that people with developmental disabilities have the capacity to be productive citizens, with many achieving independence or at least some independence. Thus, state law provides various inpatient and outpatient services for such persons. MHPs aid in the provision of evaluation and treatment services for these individuals.

What Kinds of Services Do States Provide to People With Developmental Disabilities?

Although each state gives authority to a state agency to establish and maintain services to persons with developmental disabilities, this same agency may not be required to provide such services. In addition, in most states, the courts do not have authority to order particular services for these persons. As a result, provision of services is heavily dependent on available funding and on the state's commitment to provide a certain level of service for persons with developmental disabilities. Some of the types of services that are typically offered include

- child services—infant stimulation, developmental day training, and special education;

- adult services—job training, teaching of work and personal adjustment skills, job placement, and sheltered employment;
- residential services—community residential care, respite care, and foster care;
- resource services—diagnosis and evaluation; physical, speech, occupational, and behavior therapy; health-related services; and in-home services;
- information about public resources; and
- training and practicum programs for various professionals.

Services are also provided to persons with developmental disabilities who are in state facilities and seek voluntary admission.

What Is Involved in the Application for State Services?

Persons who are competent (see chap. 5) or their guardians who are residents of the state may apply for developmental disability services. If the applicant is a minor, the child's parent or guardian completes the application. In some states, a minor over a certain age (e.g., 14 years old) may be able to complete the application if the minor is legally deemed capable of giving consent (e.g., an emancipated minor; see chap. 2).

The application usually also requires medical and psychological documentation of the person's developmental disability as well as an evaluation. An evaluation generally consists of an interview with the client or consumer and a review of his or her medical and program histories, and culminates in the evaluation team's recommending an assignment of the person to a specific program or services.

What Is Involved in the Provision and Termination of State Services?

Placement is subject to the availability of resources, and the applicant may be placed on a waiting list before certain programs and services become available. A client's placement must be reviewed periodically (e.g., every 6 months) and may result in termination of services, transfer to another program, or additional services. A client or his or her guardian may administratively appeal the proposed change or request termination of services. The state agency responsible for the service provision may automatically terminate services to a minor at age 18 unless the responsible person files a written application for the continuation of services.

What Rights Do People With Developmental Disabilities Have?

Some states have laws that specifically provide rights for persons with developmental disabilities. One state, for example, provides that no such person may be presumed incompetent, discriminated against, or deprived of any constitutional or legal right (e.g., the right to vote, practice a religion, receive services in the least restrictive setting, and have an individualized treatment plan) solely because the individual is receiving state services. Furthermore, persons with developmental disabilities living in any state facility have the right to

- not be subjected to corporal punishment (i.e., punishment inflicted on the body);
- not be administered any medication except on written authorization by a physician;
- not be physically or chemically restrained or isolated except under strict regulations in emergency situations in which the person poses a risk of danger to self, others, or property;
- not be subjected to shock treatment, psychosurgery, sterilization, or research without the informed consent of the person or the person's guardian or guardian *ad litem*; in some states, such procedures may also require court approval;
- receive and send unopened mail;
- receive private visitations;
- have private telephone conversations;
- have reasonable opportunities for interaction with the opposite sex;
- receive confidential handling of personal and medical records;
- be given a nutritionally adequate diet and regular and sufficient medical care;
- be given an education appropriate to the person's age and abilities if between the ages of 5 and 18 years old; and
- receive services that are designed to maximize their developmental potential.

VICTIMS OF DOMESTIC VIOLENCE

Some states have enacted laws that provide services, including those of MHPs, for victims of crimes, including the crime of domestic violence. For example, victim assistance boards and victim–witness programs help victims put their lives back in order after the crime and help them to testify at trial. The law generally does not mandate a role for MHPs in these programs. However, the agency responsible for these programs and services (e.g., a state or county district attorney's office) may retain MHPs to provide counseling to victims.

How Are Domestic Violence Cases Initiated?

Any person, including an MHP, may report to a law enforcement agency that domestic violence has occurred. Reporting domestic violence is not mandatory, unlike in child abuse situations (see chap. 3). Police officers may arrest a person without a warrant if the domestic violence offense is committed in their presence or if they have probable cause to believe the alleged abuser committed a crime (e.g., assault and battery). Police officers who respond to calls involving domestic violence complaints may be required to, or at least encouraged to, provide the alleged victim with information about services (e.g., hotlines and the phone numbers of local shelters).

MHPs may also identify an abusive or battering relationship, encourage victims and survivors to obtain civil or criminal orders to stop the abuse, and help clients to develop safety plans for their and their children's safety. Victim advocates, some of whom are MHPs, are especially important in domestic violence cases because survivors may be reluctant to press charges or later testify for a variety of reasons (e.g., they fear for their safety; the alleged abuser apologizes; or they need the alleged abuser's financial support). Advocates can help abused spouses seek a legal remedy.

How Can Domestic Violence Victims Be Protected?

The law provides specific protection to those persons who have been victimized and abused in a family or dating situation. For example, abused people may obtain temporary restraining orders against their alleged abusers. These orders may include requiring the accused person to vacate the house, awarding temporary custody of children to the abused partner, or requiring the alleged offender to stay away from the abused partner. MHPs may also assist the victims, as well as law enforcement, by providing education and otherwise working to further the client's best interests. Sometimes accompanying clients during the legal process may be appropriate and therapeutic.

VICTIMS OF OTHER CRIMES

In addition to services for victims of domestic violence (see the previous section), some states have enacted laws that provide benefits, services, and rights to victims and witnesses of other crimes. MHPs may become involved with the evaluation and treatment of these persons so that they can successfully participate in the prosecution of the offender as well as effectively deal with the psychological and financial sequelae of the crime.

What Services Do Victim–Witness Programs Provide?

Victim assistance boards and victim–witness programs help victims by providing a variety of services. They may help the victim or witness testify in court or assist the victim in preparing statements to the court for consideration during the offender's sentencing. They may help victims file for monetary compensation (see the next section) or obtain mental health assistance. Although some states authorize counseling programs for victims, other states do not mandate specific roles for MHPs, and thus many victim assistance personnel are unlicensed lay counselors. Finally, law enforcement and other personnel who interact with victims may be required to receive training on responding to the needs of victims and education regarding available services for victims.

May Victims Be Compensated for Their Injuries?

Some states provide that if the offender is found guilty, the court, as part of its sentence, may require that the offender pay restitution to the victim. Such restitution may be in money or required labor to benefit the victim.

Victims of certain crimes (e.g., sexual assault, kidnapping, and aggravated burglary) may also apply in some states for limited compensation even if the perpetrator is not prosecuted or convicted. This compensation may cover loss of earnings as well as medical, hospital, nursing, physical, and mental health care costs that are incurred as the result of being victimized. For example, one state provides that benefits and services available to employees under workers' compensation laws may be extended to innocent victims of criminal acts that resulted in bodily injury.

Some of these states require victims to apply to the courts, whereas others require applications to a specified state agency or a victim compensation board. Compensation may be reduced by the amount of any public or private insurance or damages obtained from a civil lawsuit against the person responsible for the victim's injury. In assessing the fairness of the compensation request, MHPs may be asked to examine the mental or emotional condition of the victim.

What Rights Do Victims Have?

The law in some states requires that criminal justice system personnel (e.g., law enforcement personnel, attorneys, and judges) treat victims with respect, fairness, and compassion as well as respect the rights of victims and witnesses of crimes. These rights may include the right to

- have access to immediate medical assistance without being detained for questioning;
- be protected from harm and threats of harm and be provided with information relevant to their safety;
- be informed as to the time and place of trial;
- be scheduled as a witness as early as practical in the court proceedings so that they can be physically present during the trial after testifying;

- be informed about and assisted in receiving available witness fees;
- be provided employer intercession services to minimize an employee's loss of pay and other benefits resulting from court appearance;
- be notified if their scheduled court appearance as a witness will need to be rescheduled;
- be provided a secure waiting area during court proceedings away from the defendant and family and friends of the defendant;
- have stolen property returned when no longer needed as evidence;
- be informed as to the time and place of the sentencing hearing;
- provide the court with a written victim impact statement to be considered during the sentencing hearing;
- present, at the sentencing hearing, a statement personally or by a representative about the impact of the offense on them;
- receive all presentence reports about the offender;
- be provided restitution by the offender in money or labor;
- be informed of the final disposition of the case; and
- present at the parole hearing personally, by a representative, or in writing their views on the appropriateness of parole for the offender.

What Rights Do Child Victims Have?

Child victims and witnesses may be afforded certain rights and protections as well. For example, one state provides that they may have the right to

- remain anonymous to everyone except to the people involved with the prosecution of the case or to the agency that provides the child protective services;
- have an advocate inform the prosecuting attorney about the ability of the child to cooperate with the prosecution and the potential effects of such cooperation;
- have the assistance of professional personnel during the interviewing of the child victim;
- have referrals to social service agencies that could assist the child and his or her family with the emotional impact of the crime and the subsequent investigation and judicial proceedings in which the child is to be involved;
- have the details of the case explained to them in easily understandable, developmentally appropriate language;
- be provided a secure waiting area during court process and be accompanied by an advocate or support person during the court proceedings;

- have professional personnel provide information to the court about the child's ability to understand the nature of the proceedings;
- have the assistance of professional personnel in court to provide emotional support to the child while the child testifies; and
- provide to the court information as to the need for other supportive persons to be present while the child testifies.

In those cases in which testimony is needed but in which the presence of support persons is not enough to ameliorate the child's emotional distress in the courtroom, other courtroom accommodations may be proposed. For example, a child who would be too emotionally traumatized to testify in front of the defendant in the courtroom may be permitted to testify via closed-circuit television. MHPs may be involved in this aspect of the case by evaluating the child and providing testimony on the need for such accommodations.

VIOLENT SEXUAL OFFENDERS

The sentencing court for adjudicated criminals may combine probation with mandated treatment for sex offenders. In such cases, the court may require the probationer to pay all or part of the costs that the victim incurred for counseling as a result of the sex offense.

In addition, some states provide specialized services for sex offenders through civil commitment to a special treatment program for indefinite periods of time. These laws are designed to protect society from sex offenders considered dangerous because of the nature of their previous crimes and future sexually violent propensities and to rehabilitate these offenders.

MHPs may be involved in evaluating these persons, testifying in court, and providing treatment to these persons. Some states require providers involved in sex offender evaluation and treatment to be certified and to be subject to standards of professional conduct unique to the certification.

What Is the Legal Standard for Civil Commitment of Violent Sexual Predators?

To be committed under these laws, the individual must have a mental illness or mental abnormality, have committed a violent sexual offense (but have not necessarily been adjudicated guilty of that offense), and have the propensity to commit similar offenses in the future.

What Is Civil Commitment of Adjudicated Sexual Offenders?

The laws also provide for the civil commitment of persons convicted of sexual offenses who have served their sentences and are scheduled to be released into the community. Under these laws, the prosecutor may initiate the civil commitment hearing prior to the person's release from prison.

How Is the Commitment Terminated?

If at any time, the MHPs at the commitment facility believe that the person no longer meets the criteria for commitment, they must release the person. In addition, the person's progress during commitment must be reviewed at regular intervals (e.g., once a year) to determine the need for further treatment. If at one of these reviews, the MHPs find that the person no longer meets the legal criteria for commitment, the person must be released.

PEOPLE IN JAIL OR PRISON

Offenders in jail or prison often have needs for mental health services either because they entered the facility with mental health problems or because the problems arose while in the facility. Some states require that such services be available because they are recognized as a vital part of the overall health care program for persons who are incarcerated. However, the funding for mental health services is often far below what is needed to provide adequate mental health care to the inmates. If MHPs' services are provided, it is typically for assessment of the inmates. Assessment information is then used by the facility administrators for classification and order maintenance purposes. MHPs may serve as employees of these institutions or in a consulting capacity.

What Mental Health Services Are Available to People in Jail?

Some states specifically provide for mental health services to detainees in jail. To ensure compliance with this law, facility personnel may be trained to recognize symptoms of mental illness and retardation and provided with written operating procedures that address screening, referral, and care of inmates with serious mental illness and retardation. Some jails provide a social service program that is administered, supervised, and run by trained MHPs to provide individual and family counseling, crisis intervention, assistance in linking inmates with existing community resources, discharge planning services, and drug and alcohol counseling services.

Unfortunately, the law in most states is not as developed. In fact, the law in some states may even restrict mental health services to certain classes of people. For example, detainees in jail who show symptoms of a mental disorder may simply be referred for involuntary civil commitment (see the previous section). If the person is committed and subsequently found to no longer have a mental disorder, he or she will be discharged from the hospital and returned to jail to finish serving the sentence.

What Mental Health Services Are Available to People in Prison?

Mental health services are generally available at all prisons, although, as already noted, the level of funding for these services may be inadequate. To try to ensure a minimum level of uniformity and competence in service provision, some states have regulations that require that a director of forensic mental health services be appointed, mental health staff be licensed, and an operations manual be developed. Such a manual might include the specification of what services are to be provided to inmates, where these services are to be provided (e.g., in a separate unit within the prison), how records are to be kept, and what procedures and rules should be followed in regard to inmate confidentiality. Because of the lack of funding for mental health services within most states' departments of corrections, inmates who show serious mental illness may need to be transferred to a special unit within an inpatient facility (e.g., state hospital) located off the prison's grounds.

Can Sex Offenders Obtain Services in Prison?

In some states, the law provides specialized services for sex offenders as part of their sentence. A sentence that involves treatment is generally predicated on showing that the person was and continues to be sexually dangerous. To make this determination, the court as part of the sentencing process may order that the offender be referred to a diagnostic and treatment center for a physical and psychological examination. MHPs may be involved in evaluating the person, testifying in court, and providing treatment to these persons as either an employee of or an independent contractor with the department of corrections.

PEOPLE WHO ARE DYING

Hospice care provides psychological and physical support for people who are terminally ill. The emphasis is on increasing the quality of a person's last days or months through active participation by the family in caring for the person while openly facing the meaning and importance of death. Continued medical assistance (e.g., using medication to control pain) is also provided so that the person can concentrate more fully on other aspects of life. A complete hospice program may consist of home care with nursing, emotional, and religious support; inpatient care with overnight services for the family; and bereavement services for the family. An MHP may be involved in all three phases as a member of the support team.

State law may regulate health care facilities operated to provide hospice care by licensing them and designating the services that they may or must provide. One state, for example, requires the following services to be included:

- nursing care;
- physical, occupational, or speech therapy;
- medical social services by a licensed social worker;
- certified home health aide services;
- medical supplies;
- physician's services;
- short-term inpatient care;
- spiritual and other counseling;
- volunteer services; and
- bereavement services.

11

LAW ENFORCEMENT

Psychologists are involved in a variety of ways in law enforcement, with perhaps the two most common law-related services being evaluation of law enforcement candidates and criminal profiling. These are important services. The first step in building an effective criminal justice process is to select persons to serve as law enforcement officers who are fit for duty. Once trained, mental health professionals (MHPs) can aid these individuals in their investigations of crimes by engaging in criminal profiling.

MHPs will also be involved in determining whether the accused is competent to waive his or her right to silence and right to counsel when talking with the police. Because these two rights typically become an issue only after the person is brought to trial, we discuss them in chapter 12. For example, it will be during a pretrial hearing that the defendant's attorney will claim that the accused's rights were violated during police interrogation, and for that reason, his or her admissions ought to be excluded from trial.

SCREENING OF POLICE OFFICERS

In some states, the title of police officer may be given to state and local police, university campus police or security officers, liquor control agents, narcotic agents, and motor vehicle division agents. State law may establish qualifications and requirements for each type of officer or the entire class of law enforcement personnel. Alternatively, the law may delegate this responsibility to a state-created council, group, or commission (e.g., a law enforcement officer advisory council or a merit system board). The law enforcement applicant must then satisfy the qualifications set forth in the law or rules and successfully complete a required training program before being commissioned as a police officer.

As part of the screening process for applicants, physicians (including psychiatrists) may administer physical examinations. Mental health examinations are also typically required and often include the administration of standardized psychological tests. Because mental fitness is often one of the requirements governing retention of police personnel, MHPs become involved in assessing or treating these individuals during training and during their careers.

In states with law enforcement councils, boards, and commissions, such groups are generally given authority to

- prescribe minimum qualifications for police officers;
- set minimum courses of training, including training related to domestic violence and rape counseling;
- prescribe minimum standards for training facilities;
- recommend advanced training curricula; and
- determine whether state and local jurisdictions adhere to minimum standards.

Pursuant to rules developed to implement these criteria, applicants are typically required to possess the following qualifications:

- U.S. citizenship;
- good physical and mental health;
- ability to read, write, and speak the English language well; and
- good moral character with no convictions for any criminal offense involving moral turpitude.

In some states, the physical health qualification must be verified by a licensed physician, and the mental health qualification must be verified by an MHP. Conditions such as personality disorders, psychosis, alcoholism or drug addiction, and emotional instability or immaturity would render the applicant unqualified. In the case of either a physical or a psychological problem, the issue becomes whether the condition or disorder would prevent a candidate from effectively performing the police officer's duties (e.g., the condition or disorder would lead to substantial loss of time on the job, early disability, and interference with job performance). Thus, MHPs should be able to demonstrate how a person's personality traits or psychological disorder would affect the police work that the person being evaluated is expected to perform.

PROFILING OF CRIMINAL SUSPECTS

MHPs are increasingly becoming involved in trying to identify typical characteristics and behavioral patterns of criminal offenders. This work may be helpful during a current or ongoing criminal investigation (e.g., profiling rapists or "school shooters"), and to develop community education and awareness projects and prevention programs. Because profiling is a law enforcement investigatory technique, there is no law regarding its use, with two exceptions. First, the use of racial profiling by police is prohibited. Although race may be scientifically appropriate for inclusion with other factors in a profile, it is illegal for police officers to use it alone to predict criminal behavior. Second, because profiling lacks an adequate scientific basis, MHPs who provide profiling services need to be aware of the way the law will evaluate whether their testimony is admissible in a court case (see the section titled Expert Witnesses in chap. 13).

12

PRETRIAL MATTERS IN CRIMINAL AND CIVIL LITIGATION

Once a person is criminally investigated, prosecuted, or civilly sued, numerous mental health issues arise. Is the accused person competent to waive his or her right to silence? What if he or she refuses counsel? Is the person competent to do so? These are issues that occur during a criminal investigation, but as noted in the prior chapter, they typically do not become a legal issue unless the district attorney decides to prosecute the person. Then these issues will be raised in pretrial motions. In addition, the judge will have to set bail for the defendant and decide whether the individual is competent to stand trial. The rights to counsel and a jury also attach in most civil trials.

Obviously, mental health professionals (MHPs) may become involved in these issues in a number of ways. When a suspect has been identified and arrested, MHPs may be asked to perform an evaluation to determine whether the defendant is or was competent to waive his or her right to silence and to counsel. A precharging evaluation may be needed to determine whether the accused person is suitable for a diversion program rather than prosecution. A pretrial evaluation may be required for the bail hearing to address the defendant's dangerousness to the community or to assess if the defendant is competent to stand trial.

COMPETENCY TO WAIVE THE RIGHTS TO
SILENCE, COUNSEL, AND A JURY

Persons questioned by police about a criminal offense that they are believed to have committed have the rights to silence (i.e., not to incriminate themselves) and legal counsel (hereinafter counsel). These rights are guaranteed under the U.S. and state constitutions. These people also have the option of waiving these rights if they are competent to do so. Finally, if charged with a criminal offense and brought to trial, criminal defendants have the right to a jury trial. The rights to be represented by an attorney and to a jury trial are not limited, however, to criminal trials. They are also available in most civil trials. MHPs may be asked to examine criminal defendants and civil litigants and testify as to whether person was or is competent to waive these rights.

What Is the Right to Silence?

The right to silence applies as soon as a person is taken into custody by a police officer. The person must be read a statement of rights, known as Miranda rights, that informs the person about his or her right to silence and that any statements made by the person may be used at trial. Until the Miranda rights are read to the person, any statements made by that person may not be introduced into evidence at trial. The accused person may choose to waive his rights and give any information requested by the police, including a confession. If a person chooses to invoke his right to silence, all questioning must stop.

The accused person must be competent to waive the right to silence, and the confession must be voluntary. In some states, confessions are presumed to be involuntary and the state must prove that the confession was given intelligently, freely, and voluntarily. In other states, confessions are presumed to be voluntary and so the defense must raise the issue of involuntariness. The court will look at the totality of the circumstances to determine whether a confession (and, by implication, the waiver of the right to silence) was voluntary. Courts have noted various factors that are important to this determination. First, a confession may not be the product of either physical or psychological coercion. For instance, in a case in which the police detectives repeatedly questioned a defendant, telling her that she would never see anyone again and that she would be committed to a psychiatric institution, the courts in one state held that her subsequent confession was involuntary. Second, evidence that a person was legally incompetent or insane at the time of the confession has been considered strong proof that the confession was involuntary. However, a defendant's mental illness or mental retardation will not always lead to a court's ruling that the waiver of rights was involuntary or that the person was incapable of waiving his or her rights.

Finally, environmental factors such as hunger, intoxication, and physical condition may be taken into account when deciding whether a waiver of the right to silence was voluntary.

What Is the Right to Counsel?

A criminal defendant is generally entitled to representation by an attorney in any criminal proceeding (i.e., felony or misdemeanor) in which a guilty judgment could lead to the defendant's imprisonment or confinement. Thus, for example, defendants who commit petty offenses such as traffic violations would not usually possess the right to counsel. Defendants who are indigent have the right to have counsel appointed for them by the state and paid for by the state.

The right to counsel is critical both in and out of trial and is part of the Miranda statement that police must read to an accused person. The right to counsel attaches as soon as the defendant is taken into custody. The attorney not only acts as a buffer against direct questioning by the police but also represents the defendant at legal proceedings. Once the right attaches, the state must direct all further communications concerning the defendant through the defendant's attorney. For example, when the right to counsel is invoked during questioning by the police, questioning must stop until the defendant's attorney is present. Questioning of the defendant without the presence of the defense attorney will likely be found to violate the defendant's right to counsel, and any information given by the defendant during this time will be inadmissible at trial.

Not all defendants choose the right to have an attorney represent them. Defendants have the right to waive their right to counsel and to represent themselves. This process is known as self-representation, *pro se* representation, or *pro per* representation. The test for whether the defendant is competent to waive the right to counsel is whether the defendant can make a knowing, intelligent, and voluntary relinquishment of the right. As stated earlier, the determination depends on the particular facts and surroundings of the case, including the background, experience, and conduct of the defendant and the conduct of the authorities.

If the defendant chooses to represent him- or herself, the court is required to advise the person about the advantages and disadvantages of self-representation. This cautioning by the court is intended to ensure that the defendant knows what he or she is doing, and is making the waiver decision "with eyes wide open."

Litigants in almost all civil trials also have the right to counsel. Although they will not become aware of this right through a Miranda warning, a court will instruct them about the importance of this right at their first appearance in court.

What Is the Right to Waive a Jury Trial?

Defendants have the right to a jury trial in felony and in some nonfelony criminal proceedings and the right to waive this right. In some states, defendants may not be able to waive this right in capital cases (i.e., cases that can result in the death penalty). The right to a jury trial also attaches in most civil cases. For example, one state's law allows for jury trials in most civil cases, including divorce actions, suits affecting the parent–child relationship (except adoptions), and personal injury actions.

In some states, the test for competency to waive the right to a jury trial is that the defendant must be able to make a knowing, intelligent, and voluntary relinquishment of the right. Other states do not use the voluntary requirement. Still other states impose additional requirements. For example, courts in one state also consider the seriousness of the crime, the complexity of the evidence, the existence of a highly charged emotional atmosphere in the community, and the amenability of the issues to resolution by a jury. If there is a substantial question as to the defendant's mental capacity, the court must make an independent determination of whether the person is mentally competent to waive this right.

PRECHARGING EVALUATIONS

Some, but not all, states provide for prosecutor-ordered mental health evaluations that are used to assist the prosecutor in determining whether to charge a person with a criminal offense or to divert him or her to the mental health system, some other social service program, or to a pretrial diversion program. Even where the law does not allow the prosecutor to require the accused person to undergo an evaluation for precharging purposes, defense counsel may support such an evaluation in an effort to convince the prosecutor to use diversion rather than prosecution.

MHPs may be involved in evaluating persons for diversion programs and in providing services to the programs as either private consultants or employees. Treatment in such programs is generally time limited (e.g., 3 years), and on successful completion of the program, charges are usually dismissed.

What Are Precharging Evaluations?

Some states have established recommended prosecutorial standards for requesting a mental health evaluation for making charging and plea dispositions. The standards may not be binding, however, and prosecutors have discretion to decide not to prosecute a case even though sufficient evidence exists to warrant prosecution.

What Are Pretrial Diversion Programs?

Some states have enacted elaborate pretrial programs that offer rehabilitative alternatives to prison. To qualify for such programs, the defendant usually must not have a criminal record, not be currently charged with a violent crime, and be amenable to treatment. Examples of other criteria that are used include the motivation of the defendant to be diverted and successfully complete the program, the age of the offender, the probability that the criminal behavior can be controlled by treatment in a diversion program, the extent to which the accused person presents a substantial danger to others, and whether the benefits to society from diversion outweigh the harm that might result from not prosecuting the individual.

BAIL DETERMINATIONS

Most, but not all, persons charged with a crime have the right to be released on bail up until conviction. Bail typically requires the posting of a financial bond that the defendant will forfeit if he or she does not show up for trial and other conditions the court may deem appropriate (e.g., avoiding contact with the victim or witness). Bail may not be excessive and is not to be imposed as a punishment because its sole purpose is to ensure that the defendant returns to court when required. When making a bail determination, the court must balance the need to secure the appearance of the accused at trial and to protect the public from new violent crimes or witness intimidation. A few states presume that bail is not required.

MHPs may contribute to bail determinations through consultation with the court or other personnel advising the court, such as police officers or probation officers, regarding the person's dangerousness, mental health, community stability, and likelihood of flight. However, the law does not require such an evaluation or consultation.

In reaching its decision about whether to impose bail, the court considers a number of factors, including

- the seriousness of the crime and the nature of the circumstances surrounding the offense;
- the weight of the evidence against the accused and the likelihood of conviction;
- the defendant's family ties and relationships, employment status and record, and financial resources;
- the defendant's reputation, character and mental condition, and the length of residence in the community;
- the willingness of responsible community members to vouch for the accused's reliability and ability to comply with the bail conditions; and

- the defendant's criminal record, past or present threats to victims or witnesses, and prior record of appearances at court proceedings.

Defendants may be released without the posting of any bond if they pose no danger to the community, they promise to appear at scheduled hearings, and a consideration of the above noted factors suggests that they will keep this promise. This result is referred to as *personal recognizance* or *ROR* (release on own recognizance).

The court may also refuse bail after considering the above factors or grant it but impose other restrictive conditions on bail, including

- placing the person in the custody of a designated person or organization agreeing to supervise the defendant;
- placing restrictions on travel, associates, or residence;
- prohibiting the person from possessing any dangerous weapon, drinking liquor, or taking illegal substances; and
- requiring the defendant to report regularly to and remain under the supervision of an officer of the court.

Failure to follow the court-imposed conditions may result in additional conditions or in the forfeiture of the bond money and in the accused person's being incarcerated pending trial.

Not every crime is bailable. For example, state law may prohibit bail in

- capital offenses (i.e., those in which the death penalty may be imposed) if there is clear proof or there is a strong presumption that the charge is valid,
- felony offenses committed in cases in which the person charged is already on bail on a separate felony charge, or
- felony offenses in which the person charged poses a substantial danger to any other person or the community and no other conditions of release can be imposed that will reasonably assure the safety of the other person or the community.

In addition, some states provide for those accused of domestic violence offenses to be held without bail because the person poses a danger to a particular person(s) or the community.

COMPETENCY TO STAND TRIAL

The U.S. and state constitutions require that the defendant be aware of and able to participate in any criminal proceedings against him or her (see chap. 9 for a discussion of juveniles' competency to stand trial). Whenever a person's competency to stand trial is questionable, MHPs may be asked to conduct a competency evaluation. They may also participate in the treatment of a defendant to make him or her competent to stand trial.

What Is the Legal Test for Competency to Stand Trial?

All states have adopted the test laid out by the U.S. Supreme Court in *Dusky v. United States* or a variant of it. A person is incompetent to stand trial if, as a result of a mental illness or defect, he or she is unable to understand the proceedings against him or her or to assist in his or her own defense.

There are two elements to this test. First, the person must have a mental illness or defect. Second, the defendant must be incapable of either understanding the proceedings or assisting in his or her defense. The second element involves determining, among other things, whether the defendant has the capacity to understand and appreciate

- his or her presence in relation to time, place, and things;
- that he or she is in a court of law charged with a criminal offense;
- that there is a judge on the bench and the role of the judge;
- that he or she has a lawyer who will undertake a defense against the charges;
- that he or she has the ability to participate in an adequate presentation of that defense; and
- that a jury may determine guilt or innocence, or if the defendant chooses to enter into plea negotiations, that he or she comprehends the consequences of a guilty plea and knowingly, intelligently, and voluntarily waives trial rights.

Under this standard, a person may have a mental illness (e.g., schizophrenia) yet still be found competent to stand trial. In addition, courts in many states have held that a defendant who is receiving psychotropic medications may be found competent even though the person would be incompetent if he or she stopped taking the medications. The sole determination is whether the defendant's present abilities and functioning allow him or her to understand the proceedings and assist defense counsel.

Because of this, all states also allow for a competency determination that is entirely independent of mental disability. For example, if a person does not speak or understand English and no interpreter for the defendant's native language is available, the person will be found incompetent to stand trial because he or she would be unable to understand the charges and proceedings and would be unable to aid in his or her defense. Finally, it should be noted that a defendant may be found "insane" at the time of the offense (see chap. 13), yet competent to stand trial and vice versa.

What Is the Legal Procedure for Raising and Determining Competency?

Defense attorneys usually raise the issue of whether a defendant is competent to stand trial after they have experienced difficulties communicating with the defendant. But the court, and prosecution in many states, also has a legal duty to ensure that an incompetent defendant does not participate in hearings against him- or herself. Thus, the court, defense counsel, or prosecution may raise the issue of competency to stand trial.

Once the issue has been raised and if the court has a reasonable doubt as to the defendant's competency to stand trial, the court may hold a hearing to decide the issue. The court may rule on the competency issue based solely on information from the attorneys and direct observation of the defendant. The court may also order a competency evaluation of the defendant. If a mental examination is undertaken, the MHP may be required to testify as to the findings, or the parties may agree to submit the matter to the court on the basis of the written reports alone.

What Is Involved in an Evaluation of Competency to Stand Trial?

If the court determines that reasonable grounds exist for an evaluation, then it will order one. In addition, the defense may also hire an MHP to evaluate the defendant and testify on this matter.

The expert(s) report will provide an opinion on

- whether the person is incompetent to stand trial;
- the cause of the incompetency;
- the most appropriate form and place of treatment, in view of the defendant's therapeutic needs and potential dangerousness; and
- when, if ever, the defendant will become competent to stand trial.

Note that the court shall not commit a defendant to a mental health facility for the purposes of an evaluation unless it determines that the examination cannot properly be conducted without commitment. Even if commitment is required, it shall only be for the period of time necessary for the examination and cannot exceed a certain period of time (e.g., 15 days).

Are Communications During an Evaluation Confidential and Privileged?

If the MHP is hired by the defense, the information obtained by the MHP is typically confidential and privileged (see chap. 3). This is not true when a criminal defendant is ordered to undergo a mental status examination by the court. Note that if a defendant has been examined to determine his or her competency to stand trial but has not raised the insanity defense, the mental status report to the prosecutor must not include any statements or summary of statements by the defendant concerning the offense. This exception precludes any attempts by the state to obtain investigative information (a confidentiality issue) or outright admissions to be used at trial (a privilege issue).

What Happens to Defendants Found Incompetent to Stand Trial?

The disposition of a person found to be incompetent to stand trial will depend on whether there is a substantial probability that the defendant will be restored to competency within a reasonable period of time. If this occurs, the court may either commit the person for up to 6 months to an inpatient facility or to an outpatient program for treatment of the legal incompetency. Commitment to an inpatient facility will occur when the court determines that the person is dangerous to self or others or that institutional treatment is the most appropriate form of therapy; otherwise, outpatient treatment is likely to be ordered.

After the person has been successfully treated for incompetency to stand trial, he or she will be returned to trial. If a person cannot be made competent to stand trial within a reasonable period of time, the person must be released, but the charges may be refiled at a later date. If the person is mentally ill and dangerous to others, the state may seek involuntary civil commitment for the person (see chap. 10).

13

TRIAL MATTERS IN CRIMINAL AND CIVIL LITIGATION

Because many criminal trials result in a loss of liberty for the defendant and many civil trials result in substantial financial judgments for the plaintiff and against the defendant, it is not surprising that lawyers seek the advice and consultation of mental health professionals (MHPs). MHPs become involved by assisting in jury selection, providing other trial consulting services, evaluating litigants, and serving as expert witnesses.

JURY SELECTION AND TRIAL CONSULTING

Trial attorneys consider jury decision making one of the most important aspects of a case. For example, the best arguments may still be unpersuasive to the jury if it is not following them or if its members are partial for some reason to the other side. Because many attorneys place a high level of importance on jury processes, MHPs are increasingly being asked to consult with attorneys on trial strategies and tactics focused on jury decision making.

MHPs may conduct pretrial community surveys, assist in constructing questions to ask potential jurors, conduct mock jury panels, and evaluate jurors on the basis of the results of pretrial surveys or in-court observations of them. Thus, MHPs can have considerable influence on whether attorneys will choose a particular juror or type of jury. In addition, if the surveys suggest that a fair jury cannot be impaneled in the locale in which the trial is being held, the MHP's survey results may be used by the attorney to argue for a change in venue (location). Finally, MHPs also serve as trial consultants and help attorneys strategize other aspects of the case.

What Are the Requirements to Be a Juror?

State law, which sets the requirements for eligibility to serve as a juror, generally includes

- age (e.g., 18 years of age or older);
- citizenship (U.S. citizen);
- residency in that state or county for a certain period of time (e.g., at least 50 days);
- mental state (e.g., not under guardianship or conservatorship; see chap. 5);
- good moral character;
- absence of felony conviction; and
- the ability to read, write, and understand the English language.

How Large Is a Jury?

The size of a jury in criminal cases varies by state and by the type of case. In general, a jury of 12 members is required in cases in which long sentences or the death penalty could be imposed. In other types of criminal cases, a smaller number of jurors (e.g., 8 members) may be permitted. The parties may agree to a smaller or a larger number. For example, a jury for a trial in a criminal arson case in one state consists of 8 persons unless the parties stipulate to a smaller number, like 6 jurors. A state may not allow juries of fewer than 6 persons in criminal cases. Alternate jurors are generally selected at the same time that the regular jurors are selected, and this may increase the number of impaneled jurors to over 12 members.

The size of a civil jury also varies by state and on the type of court in which a case is heard. In general, larger juries are required in courts with broader jurisdiction (e.g., state district courts have larger juries than county and justice courts). For example, in one state a jury for a trial in a civil case consists of 8 to 12 persons unless it is held in county, municipal, or justice court where it consists of approximately 6 persons. The parties may agree to a smaller or a larger number.

Does the Jury Have to Make a Unanimous Decision?

As a general rule, criminal trials require unanimous verdicts. Some states permit the parties and the court to stipulate that a smaller majority is sufficient (e.g., 9 of the 12 jurors). Whereas criminal trials require unanimous verdicts, civil matters do not. For example, a concurrence of 10 of the 12 jurors or 5 of the 6 jurors may be all that is needed for a verdict. Some states permit the parties to stipulate that a smaller majority is sufficient (e.g., 4 of the 6 jurors).

What Happens in Voir Dire?

The jury selection process begins by a random selection of names from voter registration or licensed-driver rolls. These persons may then be required to complete a juror eligibility questionnaire. Eligible jurors are then randomly selected to come to the courthouse when a trial or trials are to start. From the panel that arrives at the courthouse that day (e.g., 250 persons), a subset (e.g., 30–50) is randomly selected to go to the individual courtrooms for potential service on the jury in each courtroom.

From this trial panel (also called the jury venire), the parties are typically furnished with information about the jurors. Although such information may differ in each state or local jurisdiction, it could include some of the following:

- names, addresses, occupations, and ages of both juror and spouse;
- employers' names and addresses;
- number of years employed;
- marital status and number and age of children;
- length of residence in state and county;
- ownership of real estate;
- extent of education;
- length of experience, if any, as a law enforcement officer;
- previous service as a juror together with designation of court and length of service; and
- what courses in law, if any, they have taken.

The court then initiates the questioning of members of the jury venire during the process called *voir dire*. The judge will identify to the venire the parties and their counsel, briefly outline the nature of the case, and explain the nature of the examination. It will ask any questions it deems necessary regarding the potential jurors' qualifications to serve on a particular case as well as all appropriate questions requested by the attorneys. The court may also permit the attorneys to ask questions addressed to the entire panel or to individual jurors. The questioning is limited to inquiries that are intended to identify which people must be excused "for cause" and which will be excused by the attorneys using their "peremptory challenges."

An unlimited number of for cause challenges may be made. The justifications for these challenges include

- being a witness in the action,
- having served as a juror or been a witness on a previous trial between the same parties,
- having an interest in the matter,
- being connected to one of the attorneys,
- being related or otherwise connected to either party in the case (e.g., guardian, employer or employee, principal or agent, landlord or tenant, business partner, or surety or one standing bail or bond for either party),
- being biased or prejudiced in favor of or against either party,
- being unable to understand or speak English, or
- being physically incapable of sitting as a juror throughout the trial.

The attorneys present one of these justifications for their causal challenge to the court. The court then makes the final decision as to whether the juror meets the statutory criteria for dismissal. After the challenges for cause are completed, each side is entitled to their peremptory challenges.

Peremptory challenges require no stated reason but are limited. For example, in a civil case, the peremptory challenges may be limited to three strikes for each side (i.e., rejection of three people from the jury venire), whereas in a criminal case each side may be given up to six strikes.

To ensure that the causal challenges and strikes are of value to the attorneys with a jury venire of 25 or more people, the following procedure is typically used. Each venire person is given a number. Person 1 is seated in the jury box unless stricken by a causal or peremptory challenge, followed by Person 2 and so forth. Attorneys for each side typically alternate their challenges with each venire person (i.e., Side 1 goes first for venire Person 1; Side 2 goes first for venire Person 2). If a party fails to exercise a challenge for that person, the next person is seated on the jury. This process continues until the number of jurors needed for the trial and their alternates are seated.

Although attorneys may be able to influence the eventual verdict at this first stage in the trial, they are only able to reject potential jurors from serving rather than select them. And given that the number of peremptory challenges is limited, they can only reject a small subset of the venire that they might want to.

How Can the Location of a Trial Be Moved (Change of Venue)?

Trials are typically held in the jurisdiction (i.e., city or county) where the matter arose or where one of the parties resides. Each side may request (make a motion) that the location of the trial be changed, if that side can show that it would be highly unlikely that a fair and impartial jury could be impaneled in that original location. Often change of venue motions may be brought because of highly prejudicial pretrial publicity in a case. Some states require a showing that the prejudicial material reached the prospective jurors. However, judges can attempt to find an impartial jury despite the presence of publicity by delaying the trial and examining additional potential jurors.

What Other Trial Consulting Services Do Mental Health Professionals Provide?

Finally, MHPs also serve as trial consultants, helping attorneys understand the progress of their case in the eyes of the jury and helping them strategize different trial tactics that may be more persuasive than those originally planned. For example, MHPs serving as trial consultants can hire focus groups to discuss relevant portions of the case and the evidence, and use that information to help attorneys plan their overall trial planning (e.g., types of experts to use and order of presentation of evidence). They also use shadow juries (i.e., a group of people similar in personal characteristics to the actual jury members who attend the trial every day) to follow the case day-to-day, and then take their nightly feedback from the shadow jury to help plan changes in the succeeding days.

EXPERT WITNESSES

Once trials begin, MHPs help attorneys in another way. They can serve as expert witnesses to assist the trier of fact (the jury or the judge when there is no jury) in two ways. First, they can help them understand disputed facts in cases in which the facts are beyond the knowledge of a layperson. Second, without addressing the particular facts in a case, they educate them so that they can reach more informed decisions in cases in which the information they are presenting on the witness stand is beyond the knowledge of a layperson.

The ultimate determination of whether to allow testimony is within the discretion of the trial court. Thus, the trial judge in the majority of the states today is best viewed as a "gatekeeper" who decides who can testify as an expert and what opinions the expert may offer.

When Can One Be Called to Testify as an Expert Witness?

Before an expert is allowed to testify (technically referred to as being admitted to testify), the trial judge must first determine whether the subject matter of the expert witness's testimony is of such common knowledge that people of ordinary education could reach a conclusion as intelligently as the expert witness could. If yes, then expert testimony on the issue will not be admitted. For instance, some courts have held that the effects of alcohol intoxication, the adequacy of warning labels, and the potential danger posed by wild animals do not require expert witness testimony. However, the courts have allowed expert witnesses to testify on the standards of care of a health care provider and on whether psychological symptoms could be related to an industrial injury.

How Can One Qualify as an Expert Witness?

A witness is "qualified" to testify as an expert if he or she has knowledge, skill, experience, training, or education regarding the subject and if that testimony would be helpful to the trier of fact. An MHP does not have to be the leading individual in his or her field to be qualified as an expert witness. In addition, the basis for the MHP's offered information will be scrutinized to ensure that it is relevant to the issue about which he or she will be testifying and that the testimony is reliable. If the information offered is based on scientific knowledge, the majority of states now look for proof that the methods and procedures used to derive that information are scientifically valid (e.g., whether the scientific theory is testable and has been tested, the extent to which the theory has been subjected to peer review and publication, the potential error rate, and general acceptance of the underlying theory in the relevant scientific community). If the proffered testimony is based on professional knowledge, then the courts look for other indicia of its reliability (e.g., conforms to standard practices in the field). For example, a representative from the Psychic Buddies Network would probably not be permitted to give an opinion on the defendant's mental state.

Will All Relevant and Reliable Expert Testimony Be Admitted?

Not all relevant and reliable offered expert testimony will be admitted. The court will deny its admission if it determines that the information would be too time-consuming, cause confusion, or create undue prejudice in the minds of the jurors. Courts are given substantial discretion in making admissibility decisions, and their decision whether to admit an expert or particular testimony is generally not overturned on appeal unless it was "clearly erroneous."

What May One Say as an Expert Witness?

Whereas lay witnesses typically may only testify as to their sense impressions (i.e., what they saw, heard, smelled, touched, or tasted), expert witnesses may testify in the form of an opinion or inference. This means that the expert may offer an opinion based on

- personal knowledge (e.g., information gathered from his or her examination of a client or the reports of other MHPs),
- a hypothetical question, or
- facts or data that were not already proven at trial or were not admissible in evidence as long as they are reasonably relied on by other experts in the field.

The opposing attorney may attempt to discredit that testimony by focusing on the inadequacy of the basis for it, referring to passages in articles and books that are inconsistent with it, or presenting a competing expert witness. Finally, expert witnesses are subject to the same cross-examination techniques that are used against nonexpert witnesses, such as proving that the expert made prior inconsistent statements or otherwise demonstrated bias or interest in the outcome of the hearing. The expert witness's attorney may give him or her another opportunity to clarify any conflicts in his or her testimony that were brought out by cross-examination.

A controversial issue regarding expert witnesses is whether they should be able to testify as to the ultimate legal issue rather than a factual issue in a case (e.g., "Is this person legally fit to be a parent?" "Was the defendant negligent?"). Although MHPs may receive pressure by attorneys to give such testimony and although the law in most states does not restrict such testimony except in insanity cases (see the previous section), MHPs should refrain from offering any testimony that requires the MHP to go beyond the bounds of his or her expertise.

May One Be Sued for Testifying as an Expert?

Only a few states provide immunity for experts based on the acts and communications that occurred as a result of preparing for and providing testimony. It will not cover testimony that is grossly negligent or motivated by ill will.

COMPETENCY TO TESTIFY

Witnesses in civil or criminal trials must have the mental capacity to accurately and reliably testify in court. Thus, whenever there is a reasonable doubt concerning the competency of a witness, the opposing counsel or court may raise the issue because otherwise the fairness of the proceedings would be in doubt. Child witnesses are generally presumed competent to testify. In some states, however, young children (e.g., those under 10 years of age) may be questioned by the judge to determine their ability to accurately relate facts and testify in a truthful manner.

MHPs are asked to aid in these assessments and to testify as to their findings. The competency of a witness is determined at the time of the legal proceeding, not at the time the person witnesses the event in question. The competency of the witness at the time of the witnessed event, however, can be used to impeach (i.e., challenge) the witness's credibility.

What Is the Legal Test of Competency to Testify?

The legal test for competency to testify at trial varies by state but usually involves the person being mentally competent, able to understand questions, able to communicate and express him- or herself to others, and able to understand the importance of telling the truth.

For example, one state's law looks at whether the prospective witness is of unsound mind at the time of trial or whether the person is a child under a certain age and appears to be incapable of accurately perceiving the facts or of relating the facts truthfully. The definition of *unsound mind* does not simply refer to a mental or psychological disorder. Instead, the test is whether the person's mental condition deprives him or her of the ability to perceive the event about which he or she is to testify or is deprived of the ability to remember the event and communicate with the court about the event. In addition, the person must be able to understand the nature of the oath or the importance of telling the truth.

How Is a Witness's Testimonial Competency Determined?

The determination of whether a witness is competent to testify is not a jury matter but is within the court's discretion. Competency questions are most commonly raised in cases involving witnesses who are young children or who have a mental illness. However, young children or people with mental illness are not automatically incompetent to testify. For example, a court in one state found a 3-year-old child competent to testify without requesting a psychological examination of the child.

The decision process may be broken down into three parts. First, once the competency issue has been raised, the court determines whether it should conduct a preliminary interrogation of the witness. Second, if there is a reasonable doubt regarding the witness's competency, the court determines whether to order an additional examination by an MHP. Some states apply a more stringent test before allowing a psychological examination of the witness (e.g., a substantial showing of need and justification). Finally, on the basis of its own questioning, any MHPs' evaluations, and the entire record, the court determines whether the witness is competent to testify.

Finally, because witnesses are frequently first questioned by attorneys while under oath during depositions, their deposition testimony may be admissible at trial even though they are no longer competent to testify in person at the trial. A deposition is a pretrial meeting in which witnesses are questioned under oath in the same manner as they would be questioned in trial. For example, an elderly victim in one case was found to be incompetent at the trial, but a videotape of her deposition was admitted during trial after a psychologist testified that she was competent during the deposition.

PROVOCATION

Criminal laws involving provocation generally provide that persons who have committed murder (or manslaughter in some states) are entitled to a partial defense or a lesser charge (e.g., manslaughter) if the crime was committed in the heat of passion because of adequate or reasonable provocation by the victim. In states that do not recognize the defense of provocation, self-defense may be used instead.

MHPs may be called to testify regarding the defendant's state of mind at the time of the offense. For example, expert testimony about a defendant's posttraumatic stress disorder that was caused by the victim's sexual abuse as a child will be admissible to show provocation as well as the lack of intent to commit murder.

There are usually certain common elements to adequate or reasonable provocation. First, the provocation needs to be conduct or circumstances sufficient to arouse the passions (anger) in the mind of an ordinary, reasonable person under the given facts and circumstances and beyond a person's control. Generally, the test is not whether this particular defendant was reasonably provoked but whether the passion (anger) would naturally be aroused. For example, words alone or an insult may not be enough to be considered adequate provocation. However, a threat with a gun or knife, or an actual physical attack may be sufficient to raise a defense of provocation. Second, the provocation must have actually impassioned the person. In some states, a third requirement is added. There must not have been a reasonable amount of time for the defendant to cool off before killing the victim, and the defendant must not have actually cooled off prior to the act.

CULPABLE MENTAL STATE (MENS REA)

Criminal law requires that the minimum requirement for criminal liability is a person's voluntary act or failure to perform a duty that caused the criminal result (the *actus reus*) as well as the necessary "culpable mental state" or "specific criminal intent" (the *mens rea*). The purpose of determining a mental state is to distinguish between inadvertent or accidental acts and those that a person performed with a "guilty mind." A very small percentage of crimes do not require a culpable mental state or specific criminal intent (e.g., illegal possession of plutonium).

MHPs are legally entitled to testify on a defendant's culpable mental state or specific criminal intent as it pertains to the elements of the charge against him or her. They may not be asked to do so in many cases because the jury is considered competent to make this determination without the guidance of an MHP's expert opinion.

A defendant may want to present evidence that his or her psychotropic medication affected him or her in the alleged crime. Defendants have been allowed to appear before juries without medication so that the jury could assess whether the defendant's mental status might have precluded him or her from forming the necessary intent to commit the crime. Psychiatrists might also be asked to testify on this issue.

The law defines the required mental state for each offense, with the majority of offenses requiring either purpose, intention, or knowledge. Knowledge that the conduct violated the law (i.e., *scienter*) may also be required (e.g., receipt of stolen property requires that the person knew that the property was stolen). There are four hierarchical types of culpable mental states:

- purposely or intentionally—a person's objective is to cause that result or to engage in that conduct;
- knowingly—a person is aware or believes that (a) his or her conduct is highly likely to cause the result or (b) such circumstances exist that a person should have known that his or her conduct would cause the result;
- recklessly—a person is aware of but consciously disregards a substantial and unjustifiable risk that the result will occur; the risk must be of such nature and degree that disregard of such risk constitutes a gross deviation from the standard of conduct that a reasonable person would observe in that situation; a person who creates such risk but is unaware of such risk solely by reason of voluntary intoxication also acts recklessly with respect to such risk; and
- negligently (criminal negligence)—a person fails to perceive a substantial and unjustifiable risk that the result would occur; the risk must be of such nature and degree that the failure to perceive it constitutes a gross deviation from the standard of care or conduct that a reasonable person would observe in that situation.

DIMINISHED CAPACITY

In some states, the criminal law recognizes the defense of diminished capacity (diminished responsibility). There are two main variants to this defense. In some states, defendants may assert that although they may have had the requisite *mens rea* (see the previous section), it was severely diminished as a result of intoxication from substances (alcohol or drugs) or a mental illness or defect. This could result in being found guilty of a lesser charge (e.g., manslaughter rather than first-degree murder) or receiving a lesser sentence. Other states allow defendants to introduce evidence of mental problems to negate a mental element of the crime charged (e.g., purposely or knowingly), which can also result in finding a lesser offense, giving a lesser sentence, or finding no guilt at all.

MHPs may be asked to evaluate defendants in these cases and provide evidence regarding a defendant's ability or lack of ability to form a particular mental state or possess intent. One state has found that defendants are entitled to MHPs' expert services when the subject matter on which the MHP is testifying is a significant factor in the defendant's case. Thus, this standard would allow even indigent defendants the right to have an MHP appointed to provide evidence when a diminished capacity defense is raised. Diminished capacity defenses may be offered separately or in addition to the insanity defense (see the next section). In cases in which insanity is not a defense, many states impose requirements that must be satisfied before courts can allow MHP experts to testify as to their opinions about the defendant's mental state. For example, one state requires that

- the defendant lack the ability to form specific intent because of a mental disorder not amounting to insanity,
- the expert personally examine and diagnose the defendant,
- the expert be reasonably certain as to his or her opinion,
- the cause of the defendant's inability to form a specific intent be the result of intoxication or a mental disorder,
- the intoxication or mental disorder be causally connected to a lack of specific intent, and
- the inability to form a specific intent occurred at the time of the offense.

CRIMINAL RESPONSIBILITY

One of the earliest contributions by MHPs to the criminal law was the evaluation of criminal defendants who plead not guilty by reason of insanity (NGRI) because of their mental status at the time of the offense. A second more recent approach to dealing with the relationship between mental disorder and criminal responsibility is the use of the guilty but mentally ill or insane (GBMI) verdict. Some states use the GBMI verdict to supplement the insanity defense (i.e., the jury can return a verdict of GBMI or NGRI), whereas other states use it to supplant (replace) the insanity defense. If found GBMI, the defendant is considered criminally responsible (guilty) for the crime, sent to prison, and is identified for special services while incarcerated if those services are provided by the state department of corrections.

MHPs regularly evaluate defendants for either the defense or prosecution and testify as to defendants' mental status and perceptual, cognitive, and emotional functioning at the time that the criminal behavior occurred. MHPs' testimony is not considered conclusive, however. The jury may reject the expert testimony because of its lack of credibility, because of counter testimony by an expert for the opposing side, or because there is competent lay testimony that repudiates the behavioral conclusions of the expert. MHPs are also involved in the evaluation and treatment of individuals found NGRI and in need of court-ordered observation and evaluation for continued dangerousness to the community. Finally, MHPs are involved in examining the person's readiness for release and conditional release after being committed following an NGRI acquittal.

MHPs can participate in GBMI trials by evaluating the defendant and presenting testimony as to the defendant's mental status during the commission of the crime and the connection between the mental status and the person's criminal behavior. Because of the relative simplicity in the GBMI approach and the relative importance of the insanity defense to criminal defendants, in the rest of this section, we consider only the insanity defense.

What Are the Legal Tests for Insanity?

Each state chooses its own formulation of the insanity defense or may not recognize it at all. Of the states that have maintained the defense, there are two major formulations of it. A third variant, the Insanity Defense Reform Act (IDRA), is used in federal jurisdictions.

A number of states use the M'Naghten test, which holds that the defendant was insane at the time of the crime if because of a mental illness, disorder, or defect, he did not know the nature and quality of the criminal act or know that what he was doing was wrong. The criminal law limits the application of this test to defects in perception or cognition and excludes defects in emotional reasoning or personality or character disorders. Some states have added the irresistible impulse test to M'Naghten. The irresistible impulse test holds that a defendant is not criminally responsible if as a result of mental illness, he or she did not have the power to choose between right and wrong. In essence, the behavior resulted from an irresistible impulse rather than an impulse that the defendant chose not to resist. Mental defects that are the result of voluntary drug use do not support an insanity defense.

The American Law Institute's (ALI) Model Penal Code test holds that a defendant is not responsible for criminal conduct if because of mental disease or defect at the time of the conduct, the defendant lacked substantial capacity to either appreciate the criminality (wrongfulness) of the conduct or conform his or her conduct to the law's requirements. Under this test, affective disorders (i.e., to appreciate) and irresistible impulses (i.e., to conform) are included in the formulation; mental problems manifested only by repeated criminal or otherwise antisocial conduct are excluded; and the in-capacity need only be substantial rather than all or nothing. Some states that use the ALI's test have eliminated the irresistible impulse component of this test.

The IDRA's test opted to model the M'Naghten language rather than follow the ALI's test, but it limits its application to individuals with a severe mental disease or defect. It also placed the burden of proof on the defendant to establish insanity.

What Happens to Defendants Found Not Guilty by Reason of Insanity?

States vary in the way they respond to insanity defense acquittals. Some states do not specify any particular outcome, which means that the person is completely free at the end of the trial unless the state brings a civil commit-ment petition against the person. Other states provide for an automatic com-mitment hearing immediately after the trial. A third group of states require automatic commitment for observation and evaluation of the person to de-termine whether the person requires commitment (hospitalization) because of his or her continued mental illness and dangerousness to the community. Finally, a fourth approach is to automatically commit the person found NGRI. Postinsanity commitments can often be for a longer period of time than the person would have spent in prison if he or she had been found guilty.

If committed, the person will be evaluated at regular intervals (e.g., every 6 months or once a year) for release. To be released, the patient needs to show that either he or she no longer has the mental disease or defect or that he or she is not a danger to him- or herself or others. Some states require the court to approve any release decisions. Patients may also seek condi-tional release to outpatient services. In this instance, the patient will gener-ally have to show that he or she no longer requires inpatient treatment, can be treated appropriately as an outpatient, will follow an outpatient treat-ment plan, and is not likely to pose a danger to self or others during the outpatient commitment.

POLYGRAPH EVIDENCE

A polygraph examination involves the use of a polygraph instrument by a licensed examiner who reads and interprets the results. A polygraph instrument graphically records simultaneously the examinee's cardiovascu-lar and respiratory patterns, galvanic skin response, and other pertinent physi-ological changes to examine individuals for the purpose of verifying truth or detecting deception in their responses to specific questions. The use of poly-graph examinations is controversial. As a result, they are not permitted in most civil or criminal courts. When they are permitted, state law regulates the licensure of polygraph examiners and the admissibility of test results.

How Can One Be Licensed as a Polygraph Examiner?

Whereas some states do not regulate, certify, or license polygraph operators, other states provide for the licensure of and set training standards for polygraph examiners. In these states, persons must be licensed to administer or represent themselves as polygraph examiners (see chap. 1).

Is Polygraph Evidence Admissible in Court?

Although most courts reject polygraph evidence in both civil and criminal cases, a few states allow judges to decide on admissibility or permit polygraph evidence to be used in civil cases to impeach a witness. Polygraph examinations may be admissible in both civil and criminal cases if there is an agreement made between the parties before the trial begins.

In this latter situation, the parties must stipulate (agree) to the admission of the results and graphs at trial. If any of the parties refuses to stipulate, this refusal cannot be mentioned at trial. Next, the trial judge must accept such evidence. If the evidence is admitted, the opposing party has the right during trial to cross-examine the polygraph examiner. In addition, MHPs who testify in such cases may incorporate results from polygraph examinations into their evaluations. Finally, the trial judge may be required to give the jury instructions about the use of polygraph evidence. For example, the judge may instruct the jury that the examiner's testimony does not tend to prove or disprove any element of the case but at most only tends to indicate that at the time of the examination the party was or was not telling the truth. Further, the judge may be required to instruct the jury members that it is for them to determine what weight and effect such testimony should be given.

May Polygraphs Be Used as a Condition for Employment?

Some states do not allow public or private agencies to require employees or applicants to submit to polygraph examinations as conditions of their employment or prospective employment. Other states have only restricted such use in cases in which the state is an employer (e.g., a state's department of mental health and mental retardation). Violations of such laws may result in criminal or civil charges. Exceptions may be made for certain positions, such as those involving national security or law enforcement.

PSYCHOLOGICAL AUTOPSY

The term *psychological autopsy* refers to an analysis of a deceased person's (i.e., decedent) mental state at some earlier time. The motivations and mental state of a person prior to his or her death or prior to the time he or she signed a legal document are frequently critical issues in civil and criminal litigation after that person's demise. For example, a finding that a person committed suicide rather than died of accidental causes may determine whether insurance benefits will be paid. In addition, some homicide cases have involved defendants claiming self-defense against a spouse accused of domestic violence. MHPs were asked in such cases to provide a psychological autopsy of the murdered spouse to give the jury a fuller understanding of the potential provocations that may have led to the killing.

Thus, MHPs may contribute in this area by providing a retrospective psychological profile of the person who has died. This method involves forming an opinion from other people's reports or clinical records.

Not all states use the term *psychological autopsy*. In addition, some states do not allow into evidence an analysis of the deceased person's mental state by an expert who had no personal knowledge of the decedent. In such states, competency determinations need to be made when the person in question is alive, rather than attempting to reconstruct a person's mental state and competence on the basis of documents the person left behind. Other states that allow such testimony view it as less compelling evidence for the same reasons.

EMOTIONAL PROPENSITY TO SEXUAL MISCONDUCT

The law and science regarding whether a person can be found to have the propensity (i.e., tendency or predilection) to commit a sexual offense is in flux. In general, courts have not allowed evidence of a defendant's prior misconduct to prove the present crime or his or her propensity to commit future abusive acts. Evidence of these prior bad acts was deemed to be unfairly prejudicial. However, the law is changing. Some states have adopted specific exceptions to allow propensity evidence in sexual molestation cases. The Federal Rules of Evidence, whose provisions have been copied by many states, allow evidence about the defendant's propensity in any civil or criminal case in which the defendant is accused of sexual assault or molestation. In such cases, the defendant's commission of any other similar offenses is admissible "for its bearing on any matter to which it is relevant." Some states have certain requirements, however, for performing and testifying about propensity in these cases (e.g., a personal interview must be a component of the evaluation).

MHPs may be asked to evaluate the defendant and testify as to their findings regarding his or her propensity to commit sexual offenses (e.g., assault, sexual abuse, or other related crimes). In civil matters, these cases may involve allegations of assault (i.e., the victim fears the offender will harm him or her), emotional distress (i.e., from an assault or battery), or negligence in protecting victims from abuse by the defendant (e.g., negligence of day-care centers and religious communities).

Because of the fear that sex offenders will have a propensity to commit further sex crimes when released back to the community, many states have enacted registration laws. Under these laws, persons convicted of sexual offenses must register with the appropriate law enforcement department on release from prison or from the custody of certain state agencies (e.g., a department of mental health) or on receiving a sentence that does not include incarceration. Registration is required so that police are aware of such individuals in the community, and in some states, so the public can be notified and presumably be on guard to protect themselves and their families. Such persons may be required to reregister at certain periods (e.g., annually). Failure to register may be a criminal offense.

One state, for example, has created a state board or agency to maintain a central registry of sex offenders so that people can ascertain whether a named individual is a registered sex offender. This board, which generally includes MHPs with experience working with sexual offenders and victims, may also classify registered offenders according to the risk of reoffending. The factors to be analyzed may include

- criminal history factors indicative of a high risk of reoffense;
- conditions of release that minimize risk of reoffense;
- physical conditions that minimize risk of reoffense;
- whether the sex offender was a juvenile when he committed the offense, his response to treatment, and subsequent criminal history;
- whether the offender's psychological or psychiatric profile indicates a risk of recidivism;
- the sex offender's history of alcohol or substance abuse;
- the sex offender's history of participation in sex offender treatment and counseling while incarcerated or while on probation or parole and his or her response to such treatment or counseling;
- recent threats against persons or expressions of intent to commit additional offenses;
- review of any victim impact statement; and
- review of any materials submitted by the sex offender, his or her attorney, or others on his or her behalf.

The risk determination affects who is notified of the presence of a sex offender in the community. In the case of the highest risk category, the police may be required to disseminate identifying information about the offender to organizations and individuals likely to encounter the offender. These might include schools, day-care centers, religious and youth organizations, and sports leagues.

BATTERED WOMAN'S SYNDROME

Battered woman's syndrome (BWS) describes the emotional, physical, psychological, and behavioral sequelae experienced by women who have been physically abused by their partners on a regular basis over a period of time. Older terminology referred to BWS as battered wives' syndrome because it only covered women who were married to men. In states with laws addressing BWS, the law generally pertains to criminal cases. However, BWS may also be raised as an issue in civil cases. MHPs can assist in these cases by providing parties and the court with education and information about physical abuse and its effects on women in long-term relationships or as expert witnesses in civil and criminal cases involving allegedly abused women.

There are a variety of civil and criminal cases that might involve the issue of physical abuse of women and BWS. Because BWS involves excessive force, victims of physical violence might become a victim–witness in a criminal action against the abuser (e.g., assault or attempted murder) or in a civil action against the abuser (e.g., a civil suit seeking financial damages based on claims such as assault or the intentional infliction of emotional distress; see chap. 4). For example, one state found that a wife with BWS could sue her spouse for the physical and emotional injuries she suffered as a result of continuous battering that occurred during their marriage. To find in her favor, the court also required that medical, psychiatric, or psychological expert testimony establish that the battered woman was unable to take any action to improve or alter the situation on her own. Battered women may also use BWS as part of a self-defense case for injuring or murdering an abusive partner.

Although state law generally forbids BWS evidence to be used to prove that the battering occurred or that the victim is telling the truth, BWS evidence may be used to help the jury assess the victim's credibility. MHPs may be permitted to educate the court about common responses to battering using the BWS format. For example, in one case, expert testimony was permitted to explain why a battered woman stayed with her boyfriend for the rest of the day after he allegedly assaulted her. Such testimony may be used to support one side of the case or to rebut the other side's argument that the victim was exhibiting behaviors that are inconsistent with being battered.

RAPE TRAUMA SYNDROME

Rape trauma syndrome (RTS) describes emotional, physical, and psychological symptoms experienced after an attempted or completed rape as well as more moderate and varied symptoms that appear while the victim is in recovery. Although RTS was developed to offer MHPs a therapeutic framework with which to assist rape victims, RTS may be problematic for courtroom use because it is not a recognized clinical diagnosis. MHPs should consider posttraumatic stress disorder (PTSD) as a more appropriate diagnosis for some of the victims in these cases.

PTSD symptoms of rape may be used to assist in criminally prosecuting the alleged rapist, in defending rape victims in murder cases, and in civil suits by the rape victim against her assailant (e.g., assault or the intentional infliction of emotional distress; see chap. 4). Thus, MHPs are often asked to assist in related civil and criminal cases by evaluating the alleged victim, by serving as an expert witness (e.g., in defending attacks on the rape victim's credibility by defense counsel), and by treating clients who have been raped and who later become involved in the case as a victim–witness.

How Is Rape Trauma Syndrome Used in Court?

State law generally forbids evidence about the behavioral sequelae of rape to be used to prove that the rape occurred, that the victim is telling the truth, or that consent (whether or not the victim agreed to have sex) was present. Thus, although MHPs in some states may be permitted to educate the court about common responses to rape using the RTS format, MHPs in more restrictive states may not testify in this way. For example, one symptom of rape is that the victim delays reporting rape to the authorities. This type of testimony may not be permitted because jurors might wrongly conclude that a person with some of the symptoms of RTS must have been raped. When this type of testimony is permitted, it is used to rebut the other side's argument that the victim was exhibiting behaviors that are inconsistent with being raped.

In addition, some courts consider the name *rape trauma syndrome* to be too prejudicial and may only allow a general description of the rape-related responses. At least one state has held that RTS is not sufficiently accepted in the scientific community. As a result, that state does not allow expert witnesses testimony about the alleged victim's emotional or psychological trauma because it would be too prejudicial, creating an aura of scientific reliability. Instead lay witness testimony is permitted.

What Are Rape Shield Laws?

A state law may also include a "rape shield" statute. This law prevents defendants from attempting to discredit the rape victim by presenting evidence about her past sexual history or lifestyle. The purpose of these laws is to refute stereotypical notions about women and particularly women victims (e.g., they provoked the sexual assault by wearing provocative clothing) that historically led to attacks on women's credibility in these cases.

CHILD ABUSE SYNDROMES

Victims of child abuse might press criminal charges, including general charges (e.g., assault) or abuse-specific charges (e.g., child molestation), and civil claims for financial damages (e.g., assault or the intentional infliction of emotional distress; see chap. 4). As part of these legal actions, there are many different child abuse syndromes that have been proposed for use in court, including child abuse accommodation syndrome, child sexual abuse accommodation syndrome, child abuse syndrome, battered child syndrome, sexually abused child syndrome, and traumagenic dynamics. Referred to in this section under the general title of child abuse syndromes, they describe a variety of physical, psychological, and behavioral effects experienced by children after they have been abused.

Although they may have therapeutic use for MHPs who work with child victims, child abuse syndromes are problematic for the courtroom because they are not clinical diagnoses. These syndromes are only descriptive models. Accordingly, they should not be used to diagnose or identify a child as abused, although they may have value for other purposes (e.g., refuting the implication that the victim–witness's testimony lacks credibility). MHPs are often asked to assist in civil and criminal cases that involve child abuse by consulting with parties about a claim, by treating children who have been abused and their families who later become involved in litigation, and by serving as expert witnesses in these cases.

How Are Child Abuse Syndromes Used in Court?

State law generally forbids child abuse syndrome evidence to be used to prove that the abuse occurred, that the child was telling the truth, or that consent (whether the victim agreed to have sex) was not present. MHPs may be permitted to educate the court about common characteristics of child abuse victims and their responses to the abuse using a syndrome format. Generalized expert testimony may also be used to help jurors evaluate the victim's credibility and explain why victims of sexual abuse may behave inconsistently, as long as the information is not likely to be within the knowledge of most laypersons. Finally, such testimony may also be used to rebut the other side's argument that the alleged victim was exhibiting behaviors that are inconsistent with being abused. However, some courts consider identifying abuse effects as a "syndrome" to be too prejudicial. As a result, these courts may only allow a general description of the child's abuse-related responses.

How Quickly Must Civil Cases Be Filed?

The law requires that civil legal actions be brought within a certain period of time after the abuse occurred to ensure fairness to defendants in such actions. But what happens if a person at the time of the abuse is not aware of his or her right to bring such an action or is not aware that he or she is indeed being abused? This can clearly happen in the case of children. In the case of allegations of sexual abuse and the repression of memories of sexual abuse (i.e., the repressed memory syndrome), some courts have been willing to extend the time period to file civil lawsuits to when the abused individual actually discovered that he or she was abused or reasonably could have done so.

HYPNOSIS OF WITNESSES

Law enforcement officials and attorneys rely on witnesses to help reconstruct the exact circumstances of a legally important event like the scene of a homicide or an automobile accident. Because some people experience stress or trauma while witnessing such events, they may be unable to recount important facts in sufficient detail to allow legal decision makers to reach conclusions about the event. Hypnosis, therefore, may be used to alleviate the witness's stress or other condition to allow for better recall. MHPs may be asked to provide hypnosis services for this reason and to testify about the procedures used for the hypnotic induction.

When Is Someone in a Hypnotic State?

Although it is difficult to prove when someone subjected to hypnosis has or has not entered a hypnotic state, it is important to be able to address this issue in court. Some states will not apply the evidentiary rules for hypnosis if a hypnotic session with a client failed (i.e., the client did not enter the hypnotic state).

Do All States Allow Hypnotically Induced Testimony?

Not all states allow hypnotically induced information to be used in court, and when states do, they may require that the MHP–hypnotist follow certain procedures when hypnotizing and gathering information from a witness. The U.S. Supreme Court has ruled that blanket exclusion of hypnotically induced testimony by the defendant violates the defendant's right to testify on his or her own behalf. Thus, some witnesses who have had their memory hypnotically refreshed can testify under this rule. Although an MHP may use hypnosis in his or her MHP practice, the MHP may not be allowed to present information gathered as a result of all types of hypnosis in court. Similarly, clients who have been hypnotized may not be able to testify as to their recall of an event. Some states discourage any hypnotically induced testimony altogether. Many states still only permit witnesses to testify about matters that they could remember and communicate *before* the hypnosis. The purpose of this law is to protect against false memories as a result of the hypnosis. The jury in turn may be unduly influenced by such testimony.

In states that have a legal presumption against admitting the testimony of witnesses who have been previously hypnotized, there are different procedures that have been proposed to allow such testimony into the proceeding. For example, in some states, the party offering the nonhypnotically induced testimony may be able to provide the court with information that would establish what the witness knew and could remember before the hypnosis took place. One way to do this would be for the MHP–hypnotist to arrange to have the client participate in a videotaped interview regarding the event in question prior to that person's undergoing hypnosis. Videotape would be better than tape recording or writing methods to establish prehypnotic recall. Another type of procedural safeguard that some states have used is having MHPs conduct hypnosis sessions using nonsuggestive language and videotaping the session(s) to allow for cross-examination of the expert.

EYEWITNESS IDENTIFICATION

The role of the eyewitness to any event is critical in many cases. The eyewitness may be a party to the action, a victim, or a bystander. Both civil and criminal cases frequently involve such witnesses (e.g., criminal cases of assaults and homicides or civil cases involving car accidents). Eyewitness testimony raises the inevitable issue of whether an eyewitness's identification was valid at any or all of the following stages: at the time of the event, during the investigation stage (e.g., at a subsequent lineup or other identifying procedure), or during the trial.

Because judges and juries may not be aware of the factors that may influence the accuracy of eyewitness identifications and render it unreliable, MHPs may testify as to the research supporting the need for the judge and jury to exercise greater scrutiny when evaluating eyewitness testimony. MHPs may also be asked to evaluate and testify about the likely credibility of the eyewitness in a particular case (e.g., how memories of the event may be contaminated by law enforcement practices).

Some states only allow experts to testify as to disputed facts in the case (e.g., whether the eyewitness had the opportunity and capacity to observe the event and make an identification) and do not allow educational testimony to teach the jury about potential problems in eyewitness testimony in general. In addition, only those MHPs with the requisite expertise on eyewitness identifications are likely to be allowed to testify on the topic. However, it appears that MHPs may qualify as experts if they are knowledgeable about the relevant scientific literature.

PORNOGRAPHY

Although it is illegal to prepare, distribute, display or sell obscene materials, adult bookstores are a regular part of the American commercial landscape. Part of the reason is that the definition of pornography varies according to local interpretation. Whereas some localities will consider certain publications obscene, others will consider them to possess serious educational, artistic, political, or scientific value and therefore be excluded from the reach of obscenity law.

MHPs may be asked to evaluate and testify on these issues and about whether such materials are considered pornographic in their community. In the latter situation, some states permit the introduction into evidence of community surveys to assess community attitudes and values about the obscenity of the materials in question.

EMOTIONAL DISTRESS AND CIVIL LIABILITY

In many types of civil lawsuits, the injury that the victim claims to have suffered is emotional distress (mental suffering or distress). The cause of the distress, the nature of the injury, and the motivations of the injuring person determine whether a suit must be part of a larger claim (e.g., wrongful employment termination or sexual assault) or can stand by itself (i.e., intentional or negligent infliction of emotional distress).

MHPs may be asked to evaluate the person who claims to have suffered the distress and to testify as to its etiology, severity, and duration. The MHP may also be asked to testify as to whether the plaintiff is malingering and whether the defendant's wrongful act caused the plaintiff's emotional distress or if it was the result of a preexisting condition as well as treatment methods. MHPs also provide therapeutic services to help clients cope with and recover from such distress.

How Can Emotional Distress Be an Element of Another Type of Legal Claim?

There are legal claims that do not require the plaintiff–victim to suffer emotional distress to prove the liability of the defendant (e.g., a suit by a plaintiff who was physically injured by a defendant's negligence). Such a suit may include emotional distress as an element of damages, however. Psychological problems that are causally connected to the defendant's acts may be considered by the jury when assessing the amount of financial damages. Thus, damages for emotional distress may be granted when there is proof of other intentional acts by the defendant, such as wrongful employment termination, breach of contract, sexual assault, and product liability.

There are other claims that invoke, directly or indirectly, some measure of emotional distress, such as false imprisonment, slander, or invasion of privacy. The damage is largely to one's emotional well-being. Although these claims do not require evidence of emotional harm to the plaintiff to prove liability, the size of the damage award may hinge on such proof.

What Is Intentional Infliction of Emotional Distress?

Under the legal theory of intentional infliction of emotional distress, many states allow compensation for vexing harassment and other outrageous behavior that causes a person to suffer severe distress. One state refers to this legal action as the tort of outrage. To file a claim, the victim–plaintiff must generally show that the defendant's conduct was extreme and outrageous, was either intended to cause emotional distress or recklessly disregarded the near certainty that such distress would result from the conduct, and resulted in severe emotional distress in the victim.

The first element concerns a societal judgment. In some states, the plaintiff must show that the defendant's conduct is so outrageous in character and so extreme in degree as to go beyond all possible bounds of decency; the behavior would be regarded as atrocious and utterly intolerable in a civilized community. For example, the behavior of a railroad crew that refused to give any aid or summon any help for a man whose limbs had been severed by their train was held to be extreme and outrageous. MHPs can assist the court by providing evidence of community standards and norms regarding what is outrageous behavior.

The second element, which involves the defendant's intent or knowledge, is a factual determination. For example, in a famous case from the late 1800s, a man known as a prankster was held liable for lying to a woman by telling her that her husband was in the street with his legs broken.

The last element requires proof that the plaintiff actually experienced severe emotional distress. For example, consider the case of a person who shot the victim's dog in front of her knowing that she was pregnant at the time. The victim suffered severe emotional distress and a miscarriage as a result of the defendant's behavior. Although some states require that a person show physical symptoms of distress to satisfy this requirement, most states do not. The determination of the requisite level of severity varies by state. One state requires that the distress be so severe that no reasonable person could be expected to endure it. Thus, courts in that state require more than showing that a person was aggravated, embarrassed, and suffered from headaches and sleep loss.

What Is Negligent Infliction of Emotional Distress?

The law also provides for protection against negligent infliction of emotional distress. This means that the defendant did not mean or intend to cause the injury but that the injury occurred because of the defendant's negligence, and as a result of the injury, the plaintiff suffered emotional distress. In addition, an individual may establish such a claim when the defendant's negligence resulted in physical injury to a third party, but was witnessed by the plaintiff who consequently suffered severe emotional distress. For example, a mother, after watching her son die in an elevator accident, became suicidal. She was able to sue the elevator company for negligent infliction of emotional distress.

However, states may limit claims of negligent infliction of emotional distress. For example, some states require that the plaintiff must have suffered a physical injury or require that the emotional distress must be manifested as a physical injury. Anxiety, depression, or other psychological symptoms would presumably not satisfy this requirement. For instance, a woman who received a false death notice about her husband from Western Union was denied compensation because she suffered no physical harm, only mental anguish.

In some states, plaintiffs can recover for negligent infliction of emotional distress under the *zone-of-danger* rule, the foreseeability rule, or other more lenient bases. Under the zone-of-danger rule, the plaintiff either observed the death or injury at the scene of the accident or was in danger of immediate physical injury by the defendant's conduct. In other words, if the defendant's negligent conduct could have resulted in physical injury to the plaintiff, that plaintiff was in the zone of danger. For example, in a case in which the defendant's out-of-control car narrowly missed the plaintiff (a father) but injured his son, the father was held to be in the zone of danger and able to collect for negligent infliction of emotional distress. In states that have the foreseeability rule, plaintiffs can recover if they were located near the scene of the injury, if they had a close relationship to the victim, and if the emotional distress results from direct sensory observation of the injury. For instance, a father was allowed to recover as a result of seeing a car hit and kill his daughter because the court found the defendant should have foreseen that the parents of a young girl might be near the scene of the accident.

One result of the increasing societal acceptance of psychological harm is that in recent cases, a wider range of persons has been able to recover under a broader range of circumstances. For example, a person in one case was allowed to recover for being traumatized at hearing over the telephone that the family dog had been killed. Even in these cases, the majority of states still require a close personal relationship, either a blood relative or other family-type association (e.g., a stepparent), to exist between the person who was initially physically injured and the plaintiff.

CIVIL LIABILITY OF PEOPLE WITH MENTAL ILLNESS AND WRONGDOERS WHO ARE LEGALLY INCOMPETENT

A person's mental status may affect whether he or she is liable under civil law for injurious behavior caused to another and whether he or she is covered under a liability insurance policy for the injury to another. MHPs may be asked to evaluate the person and testify as to that person's mental status when the injury occurred and at the time of trial.

Can People Who Are Mentally Ill or Legally Incompetent Be Held Civilly Liable for Their Actions?

In many states, persons who are legally incompetent (see chap. 5) or mentally ill are still civilly responsible for injuries they cause to others or to property. For example, persons who have a mental disorder that prevents them from either seeing the consequences of their actions or knowing that they are wrong or dangerous will still be civilly liable. Thus, there is no insanity defense in civil cases. For instance, the court in one state decided the case of a man with schizophrenia who did not take his scheduled dose of antipsychotic medication, became psychotic, and damaged his landlord's property. The man was found grossly negligent for his actions, and as a result, was subject to summary eviction. In another state, a man who was mentally ill was held civilly liable for assaulting a fellow inmate with a knife.

Does Liability Insurance Cover the Acts of People Who Are Mentally Ill or Legally Incompetent?

Insurance policies routinely contain exclusionary clauses that deny coverage for personal injuries or property damage that were intentionally caused by the insured. Such exclusions may also extend to the costs of legal representation. For instance, automobile insurers have the right to exclude intentional acts from liability coverage. Thus, the insured person's intent becomes critical. If there is no intent to get into an accident, then the insurance policy will cover the damages.

It is difficult to determine whether a person's actions are intentional when he or she has a mental illness. As a result, a state may have enacted a legal test to make this determination. For example, one state requires proof that at the time of the act (a) the person had a mental problem; (b) the disorder deprived the person of the capacity to act in accordance with reason; and (c) the person acted on an irrational compulsion while in that condition. If all three prongs are met, the insured's conduct could not be characterized as intentional under the law, and he or she would be covered by his or her liability policy in that state.

14

POSTTRIAL CRIMINAL MATTERS

Once a criminal trial is concluded and the defendant is found guilty, other legal issues remain. These include the competency of the defendant to be sentenced; the actual sentencing hearing; the disposition, including the possibility of probation; the competency of the defendant to serve his or her sentence; parole determinations; and the competency of the defendant to be executed if a capital sentence was imposed.

Mental health professionals (MHPs) are often asked to evaluate the defendant and testify as to the defendant's continuing dangerousness, likelihood of success if placed on probation, and competency to participate in the legal and correctional processes. In addition, MHPs may become involved in providing services to defendants either on probation, serving their sentence, or on parole.

COMPETENCY TO BE SENTENCED

Even though a criminal defendant may have been competent to stand trial, he or she may not be competent to be sentenced during the sentencing phase. Just as with competency to stand trial (see chap. 12), state law generally provides that criminal defendants may not be sentenced while they are unable to understand the proceedings against them or assist in their own defense as a result of mental illness, and typically the same procedures will apply.

SENTENCING

After the court finds a defendant is guilty of a crime and that the defendant is competent to be sentenced, it may request that the defendant undergo a mental health examination before it reaches a sentencing decision. The purpose of this examination is to determine whether it is appropriate to sentence the guilty defendant to a penal institution. This information functions as a supplement to the presentencing report by a probation officer. This report includes all aspects of the defendant that may be relevant to sentencing, including the defendant's mental health history. Defendants may also hire an MHP to provide a separate evaluation.

What Is a Presentencing Mental Health Examination?

In many states, the court may order a mental health examination in any case to help it determine the most appropriate sentence for the offender. Some states limit the court's right to order such an examination to cases in which the court has discretion over the penalty, including the type of sentence (probation vs. incarceration), term of imprisonment, or amount of fine.

After the court receives the mental health examination report from the MHP, the parties must be given an opportunity to examine it. The court may then proceed directly to sentencing, may order a presentencing hearing, or may hold a presentencing conference to expedite the presentencing hearing. The presentencing hearing may be mandatory in some states if a party requests it. At that hearing, a party may introduce any reliable, relevant evidence, including that from the party's own MHP, that shows aggravating circumstances (e.g., was involved in organized criminal activity or committed the offense in an especially cruel, depraved manner) or mitigating circumstances (e.g., acted under strong provocation; had no prior criminal history; or imprisonment would constitute excessive hardship). These circumstances may be used to explain why a certain sentence should or should not be imposed or to correct or support any presentencing reports from the probation office.

The court may also desire more detailed information about the defendant's mental condition than was provided in the initial presentencing evaluation. If so, the court may commit or refer the defendant to the custody of any diagnostic facility so that another mental health evaluation can be performed. The commitment or referral usually must be limited to a certain period of time (e.g., not to exceed 90 days). Alternatively, referrals may be made to outpatient facilities.

What Happens to the Mental Health Professional's Presentencing Report?

The MHP must submit his or her report to the court a certain time before the sentencing of the defendant. As just noted, the court will then grant access to the report or a part of the report to the attorneys for the defense and prosecution. For reasons of fairness, the same material must be provided to both parties. The court may have the authority to take certain information out of the presentencing reports, such as

- diagnostic opinions that may seriously disrupt the defendant's program of treatment or rehabilitation,
- the summary and recommendations of a probation officer,
- the sources of information (e.g., third parties interviewed) obtained on a promise of confidentiality, and
- information that would disrupt an existing police investigation.

After sentencing, all diagnostic, mental health, and other presentencing reports (except for the portions excised by the court) are provided to the persons or organizations that have direct responsibility for the custody, rehabilitation, treatment, and release of the defendant. In addition, mental health reports that are prepared for presentencing hearings are usually considered matters of public record, but the court has the authority to restrict outside access to them. Finally, the court will not allow presentencing reports or any statements made in conjunction with their preparation to be used in any new proceeding concerning the defendant's guilt. If the defendant is convicted in a subsequent case, however, the presentencing reports in their unexcised form may be used for sentencing in that new case.

How Do Dangerous Offender Laws Affect Sentencing?

In some states, the sentencing law provides for increasing the term of imprisonment for defendants who pose special risks or for those who are determined to be dangerous offenders because of a propensity for future criminal activity. The legal determination of whether a defendant fits this category may depend on psychological characteristics, which could be assessed by an MHP. In other states, however, the law does not include references to psychological considerations. For example, one state bases its determination of dangerousness on whether the offense involved the use of a deadly weapon and whether the defendant had a criminal record.

How Do Habitual Offender Laws Affect Sentencing?

In some states, the criminal sentencing law provides for increasing the term of imprisonment for defendants who are likely to commit future offenses. This is determined in some states by an evaluation of the offender's psychological characteristics, which could be assessed by an MHP. In other states, however, the law pertaining to habitual offenders does not include references to psychological considerations. Other states use the "three strikes" law in which an individual convicted of a third offense and whose sentences for the previous two offenses were over a certain time period (e.g., 3 years or more) will automatically receive the maximum penalty for the third and subsequent convictions.

PROBATION

As an alternative to incarceration, a court may place a defendant on probation following his or her conviction. Probation is the placement of the defendant outside of prison for a stated amount of time while the defendant's sentence is suspended. During this period, the defendant continues under the court's jurisdiction and supervision. This means that if the defendant does not follow the terms of probation, the court may revoke the probation and reimpose the original sentence. An MHP's presentencing report may be particularly helpful to a judge in determining the appropriateness of probation and the configuration of that probation for the defendant.

Who May Qualify for Probation?

Probation is generally viewed as valuable in cases in which there is a reasonable likelihood that the defendant can be rehabilitated through the conditions of probation and will be unlikely to commit a crime once probation is completed. To increase the probability that probation will be effective, some states restrict the option of probation to certain types of cases. For example, one state allows defendants to be eligible for probation only if the defendant was not previously convicted of a felony and the maximum punishment assessed was 10 years or fewer.

What Conditions May Be Imposed During Probation?

Terms of probation generally include obeying all laws, maintaining employment, and avoiding harmful persons, places, and things. Based in part on the information presented in the presentencing investigation (see previous section), the court may also impose specific rehabilitative conditions on the defendant's probation. For example, special conditions such as counseling by an MHP and inpatient or outpatient treatment may be imposed. MHPs who supervise programs with probationers may be required to make periodic reports about the defendants' progress to the court and probation officer or office. The defendant also may be placed on supervised probation in which he or she must regularly report to a probation officer and pay a monthly fee to the court or perform unpaid community service if the defendant is indigent. As part of this, the probation officer may impose regulations that are necessary to implement the court-imposed conditions. Finally, the probation officer may modify regulations that he or she has imposed; likewise, the court may modify any condition or regulation as well as grant absolute discharge. In some states, a hearing is required to revoke or modify probation terms.

COMPETENCY TO SERVE A SENTENCE

The law in several states provides that a criminal defendant who has already been sentenced must be competent to serve that sentence. This issue typically arises in the following ways. First, if the defendant–inmate wants to pursue a posttrial appeal but is unable to do so because of a mental illness, he or she would probably undergo a mental competency hearing as described in the section on Competency to Stand Trial (see chap. 12). Second, if the defendant–inmate was not pursuing an appeal but had a severe mental illness, correctional staff aware of the problem could initiate mental health services or the inmate could apply for mental health services in prison or for a transfer to a mental health facility outside of the prison. Third, some states recognize that imprisonment may be an excessive hardship for certain inmates. For example, one state allows its courts to review the postconviction effects of imprisonment on an inmate's physical and mental health. A court may decide to release an inmate with illness or infirmity after weighing the inmate's health needs against the need for public safety and security. MHPs may participate in such determinations by evaluating inmates, testifying at transfer hearings, and providing treatment services.

PAROLE DETERMINATIONS

Parole is the conditional release of an inmate from imprisonment that entitles the inmate–parolee to serve the remainder of his or her sentence outside of prison. It differs from probation because the convicted person must first serve a period of time in a prison or other correctional facility.

Although parole determinations are generally made by a state parole board based on information supplied to it by the state department of corrections (DOC), MHPs may be asked to provide information for the parole hearing about the parolee's continuing propensity for dangerousness. Such MHPs may or may not be employed by the state DOC or parole board.

What Is a Parole Board?

Parole boards consist of a number of persons (e.g., 5 or 18) with appropriate professional or educational qualifications (e.g., degrees in law, criminal justice, or sociology), who are appointed by the governor. MHPs may serve as parole board members. Boards in some states may employ hearing officers who conduct hearings and make recommendations to the board.

The board has the exclusive power to pass on and recommend paroles, reprieves, commutations, and pardons. A court usually will not overturn the board's decision unless there is a showing that the board exceeded its authority. Although the board provides its recommendations to the governor regarding reprieves, commutations, and pardons, only the governor may grant these actions.

When Is an Inmate Eligible for Parole?

Before inmates may request parole or absolute discharge, the head of the DOC typically must certify the inmate to be eligible for parole. Certification may depend on the inmate's criminal history, his or her current sentence, and his or her record while in prison. For example, in some states, persons who are found to be dangerous and repetitive offenders may need to serve more of their sentence than other offenders do (e.g., two thirds as compared with one half of their sentence).

What Conditions May Be Imposed on Parole?

An inmate who is certified by the DOC as eligible for parole must be released if the board finds that the inmate will be likely to obey the law when released from custody. Some states also require that satisfactory employment and other stabilizing conditions be available for the inmate when released. Parole officers can assist the parolee in obtaining employment, education, or vocational training as well as in meeting other obligations. To ensure that the best interests of the inmate and the community are served, the board may impose any conditions on the inmate's parole that it deems appropriate, including

- participation in a rehabilitation program or counseling,
- attendance at regular meetings with a parole officer,
- performance of community service work,
- payment of full or partial restitution to the victim(s), and
- commitment to the state hospital for all or part of the parole period.

Violation of the parole conditions may lead to the inmate–parolee's reincarceration. A parole revocation hearing may be required after the inmate is returned to prison.

May the Parole Board Grant an Absolute Discharge?

The board in some states has the power to issue an absolute discharge from imprisonment if it finds that the inmate will live and remain at liberty without violating the law and that the discharge is not incompatible with the welfare of society. Thus, the inmate will be released without any of the previously listed conditions.

COMPETENCY TO BE EXECUTED

In states that have the death penalty, a person who has been convicted of a crime (e.g., murder) and sentenced to death must be legally competent at the time of execution. The execution of prisoners who are incompetent at the time of the execution violates the U.S. Constitution's Eighth Amendment's ban on cruel and unusual punishment because it is inhumane to execute an individual who is insane, undercuts the deterrent effect of capital punishment, and undercuts the retributive effect of the punishment. The practical purpose of this law is to prevent the execution of persons who are unable to present postconviction appeals because of mental illness. MHPs will be asked to evaluate the inmate and testify as to their findings.

Prison personnel typically must notify the county attorney of the county in which the inmate is located if there is reason to believe that the inmate is incompetent to be executed. If state law does not specify the legal standard for "competency to be executed," MHPs involved in evaluating these persons will typically rely on the test for competency to stand trial (see chap. 12): The defendant, because of a mental illness or defect, must be incapable of either understanding the proceedings or assisting in his or her defense.

Inmates who are incompetent to be executed will be committed for treatment until their competency is restored. When the defendant–inmate's competency has been restored, this fact is submitted to the governor, who then sets a new execution date.

15

WORKPLACE-RELATED SERVICES

MENTAL STATUS OF LICENSED PROFESSIONALS

State laws governing the licensure of professionals often include provisions regarding mental status. Mental health professionals (MHPs) may be asked to evaluate and testify before a licensure board or a court concerning these other professionals' mental status and its effect on their job performance as well as provide treatment to impaired professionals.

What Are the Possible Causes of Professional Incompetency That Concern the Law?

Licensed persons must be competent to perform their jobs. Incompetency can result from a lack of training, physical illness, mental illness, or alcohol or substance abuse. For example, a nurse with paranoid schizophrenia who was not taking her medication might not be able to interact rationally with patients and coworkers.

What Are the Possible Consequences of Incompetency?

Almost all state licensure laws contain provision for sanctioning incompetent professionals. The most drastic of these approaches is to revoke the person's license. For example, licensure law may specifically provide for licensure revocation if the professional is adjudicated insane or mentally incapacitated.

As a less drastic alternative, some licensure boards have established formal programs to assist impaired members of their profession and have the legal authority to order a professional to obtain treatment as a condition of continued, reinstated, or renewed licensure. Such programs are particularly valuable if impairment is due to alcohol or substance abuse. Boards may monitor a professional's progress during the treatment and rehabilitation processes.

Do All Professions Focus on Mental Status?

Not all licensure laws specifically mention mental status. For example, one state's licensure laws specifically mention mental status in the following professions: attorneys, dentists, pharmacists, physical therapists, physicians, psychiatric nurses, and psychologists, but not other licensed professionals. However, even if not specifically mentioned in a profession's licensure law (e.g., in architecture, engineering, and hairstyling), mental competency may still be implicitly required as part of licensure law and could be used to suspend or revoke a license.

COMPETENCY TO CONTRACT

Individuals wishing to buy or sell personal (e.g., cars and stereos) or real (i.e., real estate) property must have the mental capacity to enter into a contract. This is a passive requirement in that everyone is expected to possess this capacity. It can become an issue if one of the parties to the contract (or that person's legal representative) wishes to be relieved from executing his or her part of the agreement. In cases of real property, a party who wishes to undo the transfer of property may contest the deed (i.e., the actual document whereby real property, such as a house, is transferred) on the basis of mental incompetency. Although we recognize that this competency also applies outside the business context (e.g., selling something to a neighbor), we thought it most logical to include it in this chapter because contracting is most often thought of in the business context. MHPs may be asked to evaluate the competence of the person and to testify as to his or her mental status either before or at the time he or she entered into the contract.

What Is the Legal Test of Competency to Contract?

The test of whether a person is competent to enter into a contract is whether a person has the mental capacity to understand and appreciate the agreement at the time it is signed. The person should know the nature, importance, and effect of the contract.

State law generally holds that contracts with a person who has been declared legally incompetent or incapacitated and placed under the protection and responsibility of a guardian or conservator (see chap. 5) are voidable. This is because legally incompetent persons are generally held to be incapable of contracting. After a person is adjudicated incompetent, the person's guardian is given the sole authority to contract on behalf of the ward unless the court limits the guardian's powers. However, just because a person has been treated for mental problems does not in itself mean that he or she is incapable of understanding the nature and effect of an agreement and of making a valid and binding contract. For these reasons, whether a court will void a contract depends on the facts of a case.

How Is Competency to Contract Determined?

The determination of competency to contract is a factual issue for the jury (or the judge if there is no jury). Thus, evidence needs to be presented to the court to enable it to make its determination of competency to contract. Although a party may present evidence of long-standing behavior indicating inability to understand the nature and consequences of a contract, the most important consideration concerns the person's behavior at or around the time that the contract was signed. Two cases from one state will assist in making this point more clear. In one case, a woman gave careful instructions concerning a deed, and witnesses who attended the signing of the deed stated that she appeared to have a clear mind. In this case, the court held her to be competent. However, in the second case, the court found a woman incompetent to contract when she paid no attention to the deed, had to be repeatedly told where to sign, and was never informed of the significance of the document.

What Is the Effect of Incompetency to Contract?

A finding that a party to a contract was incompetent does not necessarily mean that the contract is void. In many cases, contracts will be upheld. For instance, if the contract was for necessities (e.g., food, shelter, medical care, and clothing), the law implies an obligation on the part of the incompetent person to pay for them unless the other party took advantage of the incompetent person's mental condition. If the seller overcharged the incompetent person, the court may find that the incompetent person is only liable for the reasonable value of the necessities. Even if the contract is not necessarily for necessities, the court will allow the contract to stand if the parties cannot be restored to their original positions; the contract was negotiated in good faith; the person had no reason to suspect the other's incompetence;

and the price and the terms were fair. Thus, in cases involving nonnecessities, courts generally will only rescind contracts if the status quo can be restored.

WORKERS' COMPENSATION AND INSURANCE

Workers' compensation law provides employees with protection against the treatment costs and income losses resulting from work-related accidents or disease. In addition, death benefits may be payable to certain survivors of employees in the event of work-related death. The employer either purchases compensation insurance or is self-insured to provide these benefits to its employees. These fixed and certain benefits are awarded regardless of whether anyone (i.e., the employee or the employer) is at fault for the injury. In return, the employee relinquishes the right to sue the employer.

In some states, the employee may elect to forgo benefits and retain the right to sue only if workers' compensation coverage is rejected prior to an accident. Otherwise the employee is presumed to have elected the coverage. Other states do not allow for such exemptions from the workers' compensation law.

MHPs may become involved in the workers' compensation process in two ways. First, an insurance company or other entity may request an MHP to conduct an independent evaluation to determine the nature and extent of an employee's injury and to testify about these findings at the workers' compensation hearing if there is one. Second, an injured employee may consult one of these professionals for diagnosis and treatment, with the costs for these services being paid for by workers' compensation insurance. Some states limit which types of MHPs may evaluate, testify, and treat injured workers for workers' compensation purposes.

What Is the Scope of Workers' Compensation Coverage?

Workers' compensation benefits are paid for accidents or diseases (e.g., asbestosis, silicosis, and diseases occurring from other chemical or X-ray exposure) arising out of and in the course of employment. Benefits are provided even if the employer was not negligent. A state's law may not cover some employees, such as domestic servants, farm employees, or ranch laborers.

In many states, the granting or denial of compensation depends on whether the injury is labeled an accident or a disease. For an injury to be classified as resulting from an accident, it must meet certain requirements. In one state, to be compensable, the injury must

- be unexpected; an injury is caused "by accident" when either the external cause or the resulting injury is unexpected or accidental; and

- have occurred within a reasonable and definite time; although seemingly contradictory, the criterion may include gradual injuries or injuries for which the result is repeated trauma; the logic supporting this result is that the repetitive events are considered to have contributed to the injury a little bit each day such that when the injurious effect finally materializes, the last trauma is considered what caused the injury.

Other states require the injury to produce an immediate result. Thus, repetitive traumas resulting from years of work do not qualify.

For an occupational disease to be an accident and compensable in the same state, it must be shown that the disease

- is a natural incident of the work occasioned by the nature of the employment,
- has a direct causal connection with the conditions under which the work is performed, and
- does not come from a hazard to which the employee would have been equally exposed outside of the employment.

In other states, the only requirement for both accidents and diseases is that the injury be an unintended one that arises out of the person's employment, which means that it results from risks reasonably connected or belonging to the person's job. However, compensation may not be provided when injury or death results from

- intentional self-infliction, unless it is a result of a mental disturbance that was caused by a work-related injury and its consequences;
- intoxication or the use of illegal or other controlled dangerous substances (e.g., drugs);
- failure to use a personal protective device despite repeatedly being warned to do so by the employer (except in emergency situations);
- recreational or social activities, except if they are regular incidents of employment and produce a benefit to the employer beyond improvement in employee health and morale;
- acts of God (e.g., natural disasters); and
- deterioration in function as a result of the natural aging process.

In all states, classification of an injury as an accident or an occupational disease is important because it is necessary for coverage. An injury that does not meet the requirements for one or the other cannot be compensated.

Are Mental Stress and Mental Disorders Covered?

Although all states cover physical injuries and diseases, state workers' compensation laws differ in their coverage of mental injuries and diseases. For example, some states provide coverage when a physical accident related to the person's employment causes psychological disease (disability). Similarly, mental stressors that result in physical disease (e.g., heart attacks and stroke) may be compensated. However, if the causal factor is a mental stimulus (e.g., high stress) and the resulting injury or disease is mental (e.g., a mental illness such as depression), the employee may be required to pass an objective test to determine whether the mental illness was truly caused by the mental stimulus at the workplace.

In some states, a person's mental problems can only be considered a covered accident or disease if some unexpected, unusual, or extraordinary stress related to the employment or some physical injury related to the employment was a substantial contributing cause of the mental illness or condition. The employee also may need to show that the work exposed him or her to stress that was not experienced by coworkers. Finally, the employee may have to meet a different kind of objective test for determining whether the mental stress caused a physical or mental injury (e.g., would a reasonable person have reacted to the workplace stress in that manner).

How Is a Claim Processed?

An employee who has been injured in an accident or contracts a disease that he or she believes is related to the employment generally must first notify the employer of the condition within a certain period of time (e.g., 90 days for an accident; 5 months for a disease). Some accidental injuries may require quicker notice (e.g., 48 hours for an inguinal hernia). Other states do not require a well-defined time limit because each case is decided on its particular merits.

The employee is also generally required to file a claim with the state workers' compensation agency within a certain period of time (e.g., 1 or 2 years). This critical period is called the statute of limitations. It requires the employee to file a claim within the time period (e.g., 1 or 2 years) following the date that the worker knew or should have known the nature of the disability and its relation to the employment. If the claim is not filed within this time period, the worker loses the right to file the claim.

Some states also require the treating professional, including MHPs, to report the injury to the employer. Failure to do so could be punishable as a petty offense. Note, however, that in practice the decision whether to give notice to the employer of the injury is typically left to the employee; the professional is not likely to be prosecuted for failure to report a job-related injury if the employee elects not to file a claim. In addition, the employer's doctor may be required to report the injury to the state agency that oversees the administration of the workers' compensation process (e.g., the industrial commission or division of workers' compensation). Last, the doctor or MHP may be required to inform the worker of his or her rights under the law and assist him or her in making an application for compensation.

Once a claim is filed, the employer will be required to file a report with the state agency or the employer's insurance company. A state's law may require the report to be filed within a certain time of receiving a report and to contain certain information (e.g., the employee's personal information and the date and description of the injury).

Finally, the administrating agency will consider the claim. If the claim is considered meritorious, the employer or the employer's insurance carrier (typically the latter) will make payment to the claimant unless the claim concerns certain permanent injuries or a death benefit award. In those cases, the state agency determines the amount of compensation. In other states, an informal hearing is held with the parties, the workers' compensation judge, and the state agency to reach an agreement on the existence of liability, and if liable, the extent of disability and the settlement amount.

The majority of claims are settled at the conclusion of these steps. However, if either party is not satisfied with the outcome, that party may appeal to the administrative agency, which will conduct a formal hearing or trial. At the hearing, an administrative law judge will listen to the evidence presented by the parties and decide the claim. If either party is not satisfied with the decision of the administrative judge, that party may appeal to the state court of appeals and state supreme court.

What Benefits Are Available Under Workers' Compensation?

Generally, workers' compensation provides the employee with three types of benefits (medical, disability, and death) that are each considered independent of the others. In addition, some states have a program to provide rehabilitation services to train or retrain injured workers.

Medical care benefits, including MHPs' services, cover immediate and long-term expenses for the treatment of the injury or disease. Nursing, prosthetic devices, chiropractic services, medicines, and reasonable expenses for physical rehabilitation may also be included.

Disability payments cover the loss of income during recuperation and are classified according to the seriousness of the injury (i.e., whether it results in total or partial loss of income) and its duration (i.e., whether it is permanent or temporary). It is possible, however, for an injury to result in more than one type of classification. For example, although an injury may initially prevent an employee from working (a temporary total condition), it may eventually subside, allowing the person to return to work part-time (permanent partial disability). The rating of the percentage of functional impairment must be in accordance with a state's law. For example, some states use the standards for the evaluation of permanent impairment as published by the American Medical Association in *Guides to the Evaluation of Permanent Impairment*. Finally, disability awards may be divided into scheduled and unscheduled benefits. Scheduled benefits concern the loss of bodily function, such as deafness or loss of a limb; unscheduled benefits concern all other injuries and require a determination of the nature and extent of the impairment.

Death benefits cover burial expenses and payments to certain relatives of the employee. The law may only cover dependent children or may include dependent siblings, grandparents, and adult children. Benefits may extend to the employee's surviving spouse and parents. Payments may terminate when the child reaches the age of majority or if the surviving spouse remarries.

VOCATIONAL DISABILITY SERVICES

A state agency administers a vocational rehabilitation (VR) program that is jointly funded by the state and federal governments. It is intended for persons who have a physical or mental disability that currently prevents them from obtaining (or maintaining) employment or attaining personal independence but who might be able to engage (or continue) in gainful occupation or attain personal independence if given VR services. Certain states have expanded coverage to those with developmental disabilities and visual handicaps as well as people on public assistance.

Only certain MHPs (e.g., psychologists and psychiatrists) may be allowed by a state's law to provide evaluative, consultative, and therapeutic services. Such MHPs are either employees of the state agency or independent contractors with the state agency. A state agency's VR department may directly employ other MHPs (e.g., social workers and counselors) as VR counselors. They provide nonpsychological and nonpsychiatric services in accordance with the agency's guidelines.

Under VR law, approved MHPs' diagnostic and consultative services to VR clients and counselors are covered as are mental restoration services. MHPs may undertake evaluations in cases in which mental or emotional disorders, drug addiction, or alcoholism is suspected. The evaluation may include scoring and interpretation of psychological tests, diagnosis of mental or emotional disorder, and recommendations for appropriate counseling, treatment, or training strategies that will help the person to become more employable. When a person presents with mental retardation, a separate mental disability evaluation that includes a valid test of intelligence and an assessment of social functioning, educational progress, and achievement may be required.

Who May Receive Vocational Rehabilitation Services?

Some states have restrictions on who may apply for VR services. For example, one state allows any person who has either reached the age of 18 years old, is married, is in the armed forces, or is living away from home and is self-supporting to apply for VR services. Any person not meeting these requirements may also apply but must have a parent or guardian cosign. States may or may not have a residency requirement.

All states have criteria that are used to determine whether a person is eligible for VR services. Eligibility is largely determined by diagnostic studies (an evaluation), which involve a series of sequential assessments, some of which are more complex than described in this chapter. As a threshold requirement for VR services, preliminary diagnostic studies determine

- whether the person has a physical or mental disability that constitutes or results in a substantial impediment to employment and
- whether the person is reasonably expected to benefit from VR services in terms of employment capability (e.g., to prepare for, engage in, or retain gainful employment).

The study may also reveal that an extended evaluation of the person's ability to be rehabilitated is necessary. This preliminary study may result in the VR counselor assigning the applicant with a severity rating and a priority category for the receipt of services.

After the VR counselor determines that an applicant is eligible to receive VR services, a thorough assessment is required to determine the nature and scope of the needed services. This second type of diagnostic study involves the creation of an individualized written rehabilitation program (IWRP). The assessment identifies the person's strengths, resources, priorities, needs, and interests. It may consist of an evaluation of pertinent medical, psychological, vocational, educational, and related factors (e.g., personal and social adjustment, patterns of work behavior, ability to acquire job skills, and capacity for successful job performance) that bear on the person's employment abilities and impairments. This assessment allows for a determination of the person's goals and objectives as well as the nature and scope of the VR services that are needed, all of which are included in the person's IWRP.

If the state agency is unable to determine whether VR services will benefit the individual, but he or she meets all other criteria, the agency may engage in an extended evaluation. This extended evaluation may last up to a certain time period (e.g., 18 months). During this time, the individual may receive those VR services agreed on by the VR counselor and the client in the written plan. The individual's progress is assessed regularly (e.g., every 90 days) as though the client was determined to be fully eligible for services.

The extended evaluation is terminated when the determination about the person's ability to benefit from VR services is made.

What Services Are Available to Vocational Rehabilitation Clients?

Once an applicant is found to be eligible for services, he or she may receive, in accordance with the IWRP, the following:

- needs assessment services;
- counseling, guidance, and referral;
- physical restoration and rehabilitation services that may include prosthetic or orthotic devices, speech or hearing therapy, or mental health services;
- mental restoration and rehabilitation services that may include hospitalization or other psychological or psychiatric treatment for mental and emotional disorders;
- job search, placement, and retention assistance;
- vocational and other training services, including books, materials, on-the-job training, and classroom education;
- transportation;
- maintenance (i.e., case payments to cover basic living requirements);
- services to members of the client's family who are necessary to the adjustment or rehabilitation of the client;
- interpreter services for deaf clients;
- reader rehabilitation teaching services and orientation and mobility services for blind clients;
- telecommunication, sensory, and other technological aids and devices;
- occupational licenses, tools, equipment, initial stocks, and supplies;
- other goods and services that can be reasonably expected to benefit a client's employability; and
- extended rehabilitation services for individuals with severe handicaps.

Some states specify certain MHP services and fees in their law. When MHPs provide individual, family, and group therapeutic services to clients, they may be required to submit appropriate reports. For example, an initial report outlining the problem, proposing services and therapy goals, and estimating time frames in which such goals will be accomplished may be required. This report is separate from the diagnostic studies and psychological evaluations previously noted. There may also be regular progress reports to be submitted at certain intervals (e.g., no less frequently than once every 3 months). State law may also provide that MHPs are required to approve any psychosocial rehabilitation programs and permitted to request authorization for additional services not specified in the IWRP.

UNFAIR COMPETITION AND TRADEMARK INFRINGEMENT

Business competitors may engage in fierce battles to control or win a share of the market for their goods or services. Although competition is encouraged in our society, some types of competition can result in civil liability if the business tactics do not serve the public interest or have been legally declared "unfair." State laws prohibit unfair or deceptive acts or practices as well as unfair methods of competition in a broad variety of matters. Some of these include defaming competitors or their goods, stealing trade secrets, or starting a business with an ex-employer's customer lists.

A large area of this type of business practice is of interest to MHPs, particularly psychologists, because it attempts to confuse the consumer into believing that one business's products or services were produced by another. MHPs may be asked to conduct research (e.g., consumer surveys) to determine whether the defendant's business practices resulted in such confusion and to testify in court as to their findings.

What Is the Legal Test for Unfair Competition?

Unfair competition involves a business's (Business 1) use of the name, symbol, label, or other property used by another business (Business 2) to induce consumers to buy a product from Business 1 because of the false belief that it was produced or backed by Business 2. In many cases, this may involve a practice referred to as "palming off." In this form of unfair competition, consumers of a good or service are made to believe that they are buying the good or service of a better known competitor (Business 2) rather than that of the lesser known company (Business 1). When this occurs, Business 2 can sue Business 1 to recover financial losses and to stop Business 1 from continuing the unfair practice. To win its lawsuit, Business 2 (the plaintiff) must generally prove that the defendant (i.e., the business accused of unfair competition) took some action to mislead or confuse purchasers as to the identity of the manufacturer of their merchandise and that consumers were misled or confused.

In some states, there are two elements in proving product confusion. First, the product must have acquired a special significance whereby the public identifies it as made or sold by a particular manufacturer. Second, the product and its characteristics must confuse the public (i.e., the public cannot tell who made the product or must be unaware that the product is a copy of the original). Courts will consider the particular facts and circumstances of each case. They will consider the form, shape, and color of the package, product, or advertising, and any pictures, words, or other labels when determining whether the similarity of the products caused consumer confusion.

What Is Trademark Infringement?

A trademark is any mark, word (e.g., a business name), letter, number, design, or picture that is used by a person to designate his or her goods. It must be affixed to the goods and must not be a common or generic name. Trademarks are typically registered under federal law but may be registered under state law. In either event, registration is not determinative of whether the person has established a trademark. The relevant inquiry generally turns on whether the mark is a generic term or symbol or has an established distinctiveness. For instance, evidence that the word *hoagie* was used in a general manner in other cities to refer to a sandwich precluded its use as a trademark despite the fact it had been federally registered.

Like unfair competition, trademark infringement is concerned with confusion of the public. If such confusion exists, the relevant inquiry for the court is whether the trademark taken by Business 1 (the defendant) had previously come to indicate Business 2's (the plaintiff's) business.

Consider this case. A defendant began a business with the name "Therapeutic Supply of Main Street" after her prior partners had been using the name "Therapeutic Supply Company." The court would probably find that confusion was calculated here. Whether there is confusion depends not only on the similarity in names but also in the types of service, clientele, and related factors. Thus, confusion may not be found if two businesses have the same names but very different business products, services, and clientele.

SEXUAL HARASSMENT

Sexual harassment is illegal and unethical. MHPs may become involved in this area by consulting with businesses and public entities (e.g., public schools) about how to avoid sexual harassment, by evaluating persons who allege sexual harassment, and by testifying in court about their findings. Unfortunately, MHPs may also become involved as a defendant in a lawsuit brought because of sexually harassing behaviors by the MHP toward another person. MHPs who engage in sex or other unwanted forms of behavior with clients, coworkers, or supervisees may lose their professional license and may be sued civilly or criminally (e.g., for assault, battery, false imprisonment, or negligent or intentional infliction of emotional distress; see chaps. 1 and 4).

The law traditionally defines sexual harassment as persistent and unwanted sexual advances made by a person(s) in a workplace. This includes the use of deliberate or repeated comments, gestures, or physical contacts of a sexual nature. There are two main types of sexual harassment.

First, quid pro quo harassment involves a person in power who requests or demands sex from a person with less power in exchange for economic or other privileges. Consider the example posed in the introduction to Part II. Lee would probably be able to bring a suit for quid pro quo harassment if her supervisor told her that the only way she would get her quarterly bonus was if she would have sex with him.

The second type of harassment involves the creation of a hostile work environment in which the person is intimidated or demeaned because of his or her gender. Differences of power are not required for this form of sexual harassment. Courts use different standards when determining whether the alleged wrongful behavior is reasonably perceived as harassment. States vary in whether they require the perception to be judged against the perspective of a "reasonable person," "reasonable woman," or the victim. Again, consider the example posed in the introduction to Part II. Lee would probably be able to bring a suit for harassment if her coworkers frequently made sexist jokes, put up posters of naked and semiclothed women, touched her inappropriately, and made demeaning and sexually suggestive remarks to her.

EMPLOYMENT DISCRIMINATION

The law prohibits employers from engaging in discriminatory employment practices based on race, color, religion, creed, sex–gender, age, national origin, ancestry, marital status, pregnancy, sexual orientation, and the presence of any sensory, mental, or physical disability. MHPs are often asked to advise employer–clients about nondiscriminatory approaches to personnel selection, discharge, and promotion. They also become involved in assessing persons who allege employment discrimination based on a mental disability and may be asked to testify in court as to their findings.

Who Is Affected by Employment Discrimination Law?

State employment discrimination law applies to employers or persons acting in the interest of an employer who employ a certain number of persons (e.g., more than eight). The law may also specify an amount of time that the employee must have worked (e.g., each working day for 20 weeks) in the current or preceding year to benefit from certain provisions of the law. In addition to these limitations, state law does not cover all employers and employees. In some states, these laws may not include

- religious or sectarian organizations that are not organized for private profit,
- federal employees,
- Native American tribal employees,

- private membership clubs that are exempt from taxation under section 501(c) of the Internal Revenue Code,
- employees who are elected public officials or appointees not subject to civil service laws, and
- employees of family members.

What Employment Practices Are Unlawful?

In general, state employment discrimination law prohibits employers and their agents from engaging in discriminatory employment practice, including

- failing or refusing to hire persons, discharging persons, or otherwise discriminating against them with respect to compensation, terms, conditions, or privileges of employment because of race, color, religion, creed, sex–gender, age, national origin, ancestry, marital status, pregnancy, sexual orientation, and the presence of any sensory, mental, or physical disability;
- limiting, segregating, or classifying employees or applicants for employment in any way that would deprive or tend to deprive them of employment opportunities or otherwise adversely affect their status as employees because of the above characteristics;
- retaliating or discriminating against employees who oppose a discriminatory practice or who file charges, testify, or assist other employees in pursuing a claim for employment discrimination;
- aiding, abetting, inciting, or coercing other persons to engage in or perform a discriminatory practice; and
- printing, publishing or distributing a notice, advertisement, or other information relating to employment that indicates discriminatory practices.

Some states, however, permit discriminatory employment practices under certain circumstances. For example, one state's law provides for

- discrimination based on religion, sex, age, or national origin if the status is a bona fide occupational qualification reasonably necessary to the normal operation of the employer (e.g., minimum or maximum age requirements may be imposed for firefighters or police officers);
- different standards of compensation or conditions of employment on the basis of a bona fide seniority or merit system or a system that measures earnings by quantity or quality of production or is based on employment in different locations (e.g., reflecting different costs and standards of living), provided that

such differences are not the result of an intention to discriminate or used to discriminate; and

- giving and acting on the results of any professionally developed ability test, provided that the test, its administration, and actions based on its results are not designed, intended, or used to discriminate.

This last exclusion requires MHPs who engage in personnel testing or employment consulting to be particularly sensitive to the validity, reliability, and use of their assessment measures. In one state, the use of the original *Minnesota Multiphasic Personality Inventory* (i.e., instead of the updated MMPI–2 or MMPI–A) was questioned because it contains questions about religion and sexual orientation that employers are no longer permitted to ask of employees. Finally, employers in some states are not required to grant preferential treatment on account of an imbalance in various categories or status and the overall percentage of those categories in the state population.

What Legal Remedies Are Available to Victims of Employment Discrimination?

Any person injured by such discrimination may file a lawsuit in civil court to stop (i.e., enjoin) further violations of the law and to recover the financial damages that the person suffered as a result of the discriminatory employment practices (e.g., back wages). The person may also be entitled to a refund for the expenses of the lawsuit (e.g., attorney's fees) and other remedies authorized by the law, including punitive damages.

VIOLENCE IN THE WORKPLACE

Violence is a serious safety and health issue in many workplaces. According to recent national statistics, nearly 1,000 workers are murdered and 1.5 million are assaulted in the workplace each year.

These numbers also include MHPs who are particularly at risk for assaults. According to the Department of Justice's National Crime Victimization Survey, MHPs are ranked 7th and mental health custodial workers are ranked 10th in the occupations most at risk for violent workplace crime. Other statistics reveal that more assaults occur in the health care and social services industries than in any other. For example, Bureau of Labor Statistics data for 1993 showed health care and social service workers having the highest incidence of assault injuries. Almost two thirds of the nonfatal assaults occurred in nursing homes, hospitals, and establishments providing residential care and other social services. Such violence may come from a variety of sources, including patients or clients, third parties (e.g., robbers or muggers), and coworkers.

Thus, MHPs need to be concerned about violence in their own workplace as well as in the workplaces of their business clients. MHPs can help business clients prevent violence in their workplace, defuse current violent situations, and provide services to employee–victims of this violence. For example, MHPs can provide assistance to employers regarding hiring practices, provide training to employees on resolving conflicts without violence, help employers set up a work environment that minimizes the likelihood of violence erupting, and help employees recover from mental health problems or other injuries caused by past acts of workplace violence.

Can the Law Help Protect Employees Against Potential Violence?

Some laws are designed to protect people from violent or potentially violent or harassing behavior by restricting contact between the parties. Consider the case posed in the introduction to Part II of an employee who fears her abusive ex-boyfriend. If he engages in a pattern of hostile and threatening behavior against Lee outside of her workplace, he might be charged with stalking her. Lee could also obtain a restraining or protective order against her ex-boyfriend, which could mandate that he stay a certain distance from Lee (e.g., one mile) at all times, including when she is at work.

Other laws could also apply. If an ex-employee who was angry for being fired from his or her job returned to work and threatened to kill his or her ex-supervisor with a gun, the ex-employee could be brought up on criminal charges (e.g., assault with a deadly weapon or attempted murder) or civil charges (e.g., intentional infliction of emotional distress or assault and battery). If the ex-employee was found to be a continued danger to him- or herself or others, he or she could be subject to civil commitment if he or she also had a mental illness (see chap. 10).

Do Employers Have a Legal Duty to Protect Their Employees From Potential Violence?

Under federal law (i.e., the Occupational Safety and Health Act of 1970), employers are required to provide employees with a place of employment that is free from recognized hazards that are causing or likely to cause death or serious physical harm. On the basis of this act, many states have adopted laws or guidelines for employers to provide safe workplaces for employees by requiring or suggesting prevention programs as well as postincident response and evaluation programs (e.g., trauma-crisis counseling and employee assistance programs). A few states limit their laws to covering public employees only.

Practical prevention measures that can significantly reduce serious threats to worker safety usually consist of four components:

- demonstrating employer or management commitment to safety and security and employee involvement to achieve this goal (e.g., zero-tolerance policy);
- analyzing workplace safety and risk factors;
- designing and using administrative and work practice controls to prevent or limit violent incidents (e.g., alarm systems, emergency procedures in case of violent incident, adequate staffing, bright and effective lighting, and arranging furniture to prevent entrapment); and
- training and educating employees about security hazards and ways to protect themselves and their coworkers.

State law may be used to hold employers liable for their actions or inaction regarding workplace violence. For example, in one state, a company may be held liable for negligent hiring practices if it hires an employee without a thorough background check. In addition, it can be held liable for negligent retention practices if it has information regarding violent acts by an employee and does nothing about it.

CONCLUSION:
TAKING THE NEXT STEP

After reading this book, a mental health professional (MHP) understands a significant amount about the law that affects his or her practice. The MHP has read about how the law provides benefits and practice opportunities and creates obligations that he or she must follow to avoid liability. The MHP also now understands more about how the law creates special concerns and benefits for clients, which may affect the services that he or she provides to them.

One final issue remains to be addressed. This book is intended to provide the MHP with an introduction to, and not serve as an advanced text on, the law affecting mental health practice. For example, the volume teaches the typical way the law works on each topic, rather than discussing the specific way the law works in each state. It is important, therefore, that an MHP take the next step and learn the relevant law affecting practice in his or her state. We hope that the introduction to the law provided in this book makes understanding state law a less daunting and more manageable task. As noted in the introduction, if one has a *Law and Mental Health Professionals* volume (published by the American Psychological Association) devoted to the relevant state, reading it will give one the specifics of what one needs to know. Lawyers are another source for learning about the specifics of the law in a state. This book will help an MHP talk with attorneys who provide consulting services and with lawyers when the need arises, in a more intelligent and focused way. Ultimately, we hope that this volume opens up new practice opportunities for MHPs and allows them to practice more competently in the future.

RECOMMENDED READINGS

Law & Mental Health Professionals Series
Bruce D. Sales and Michael Owen Miller, Series Editors

ALABAMA: Bentley, Reaves, and Pippin
ARIZONA, 2ND ED.: Miller, Sales, and Delgado
CALIFORNIA: Caudill and Pope
CONNECTICUT: Taub
DELAWARE: Britton and Rohs
FLORIDA, 2ND ED.: Petrila and Otto
GEORGIA: Remar and Hubert
KENTUCKY: Drogin
MASSACHUSETTS, 2ND ED.: Brant
MICHIGAN: Clark and Clark
MINNESOTA: Janus, Mickelson, and Sanders
NEVADA: Johns and Dillehay
NEW JERSEY, 2ND ED.: Wulach
NEW YORK: Wulach
NORTH DAKOTA: O'Neill and Lochow
OHIO: VandeCreek and Kapp
PENNSYLVANIA: Bersoff, Field, Anderer, and Zaplac
SOUTH CAROLINA: Follingstad and McCormick
SOUTH DAKOTA: Cichon
TEXAS, 3RD ED.: Shuman
VIRGINIA: Porfiri and Resnick
WASHINGTON: Benjamin, Rosenwald, Overcast, and Feldman
WISCONSIN: Kaplan and Miller
WYOMING: Blau

INDEX

assault and battery and, 65
negligent homicide and, 65
sexual offenses and, 64
Criminal liability, 64–65
Criminal negligence, 176
Criminal responsibility
guilty but mentally ill or insane, 177
not guilty by reason of insanity and, 177
Criminal trials
jury size in, 168
unanimity in, 169
Criminal *vs.* civil action, liability and, 62
Culpable mental state (mens rea)
in criminal liability, 175
types of, 176
Custodial interference, defined, 28
Custody
in child abuse and neglect, 103
of juvenile by court, 123
temporary in child abuse, 101
criteria for, 102
preliminary hearing for, 102

Dangerous offender laws, 195
Dangerous persons, confidentiality and, 41–42
Danger to community, juvenile, court placement in, 125
Danger to self or other
commitment release and, 179
emergency commitment for, 135
emergency treatment for alcoholism and, 138–139
involuntary commitment for, 165
Defamation of character, civil liability for, 62–63
Delinquent children, defined, 122
Dependency hearing, 102
Dependent children, defined, 122
Deposition, 78, 174–175
Developmental disabilities
defined, 143
placement for, 144
Developmental disabilities, persons with. *See also* Disability services
application, provision, termination of state services for, 143–144
state services for, 143–144
Diminished capacity. *See also* Capacity
Diminished capacity defense
in criminal law, 176–177
requirements for, 177

Disability services. *See also* Developmental disabilities, persons with
vocational, 208–211
Diversion programs
pretrial, 161
vs. prosecution, 157
Divorce
fault grounds for, 116
irreconcilable differences or irreparable break in marriage, 115–116
mediation and, 115
no fault, 115
outcome of, 116
petition to court for, 115
procedure to obtain, 115–116
summary-disposition procedure in, 117
temporary child support or spousal maintenance, 116
Domestic violence
bail and, 162
initiation of cases, 145–146
protection of victims of, 146
victim advocates and, 146
Driver's license
compensated disability and, 76
denial, suspension, revocation of, 75–76
disqualification for, 75, 76
reasonable accommodation for qualified disabled persons and, 76
Drug abuse, testamentary capacity and, 80
Drug treatment courts (DTCs)
admission criteria for, 142
defined, 141
duration of treatment in, 142–143
elements of, 141
interventions in, 142
origin of, 140–141
participation in, 142
planning and funding of, 141
relapse and, 143
routes to, 142
Duty to assess, for potential violence, 41
Duty to protect
from dangerous persons, confidentiality and, 40–41
discharge of, 41
as exception to confidentiality, 41
from violence in the workplace, 216
Dying persons, hospice care for, 151

Education, for licensure, 16

Self-representation, waiver of right to counsel and, 159
Senility, testamentary capacity and, 80
Sentencing
    competency and, 193–194, 197
    dangerous offender laws and, 195
    habitual offender laws and, 195–196
    presentencing mental health examination and, 194
    report of presentencing mental health examination and, 195
Sex offenders, mental health services for in prison, 151
Sexual harassment
    defined, 212
    hostile work environment as, 213
    loss of professional license for, 212
    quid pro quo, 213
Sexual misconduct
    determination of reoffence and, 182
    emotional propensity to, 181
    registration laws and central registry of offenders, 182
Sexual offenders. *See also* Violent sexual predators
    civil commitment of, 149–150
    specialized services for, 149
Sexual offenses
    with mentally disordered person, 64
    sexual contact or intercourse without consent, 64
Shadow jury, 171
Silence, right to, 158–159
Slander, 62
Special education
    for children with disabilities and special needs, 107, 110–112
    for gifted and talented children, 107–109
Staff privileges
    defined, 14
    description of, 20–21
    regulation of, 21
Standards of care, malpractice suits and, 53, 55, 56
State law, sources of, 5
State licensure boards, complaints before, 65–66
State professional ethics committees, complaints before, 65–66
Subpoena
    contempt of court and, 48

defined, 34, 47
    putting into effect, 47–48
Substance abuse. *See also* Drug treatment courts (DTCs)
    biopsychosocial approach to, 141
    defined, 141
    drug courts for persons with, 140–143
    insurance coverage for, 32
Substituted judgment, in abortion decision, 87
Suicide or suicidality, testamentary capacity and, 80
Sunset
    of credentialing agencies and regulations, 20
    defined, 14
Supervisee, responsibilities of, 21
Supervision
    persons in need of, defined, 122
    supervisee responsibilities in, 21
    supervisor responsibilities in, 22
Supervisor
    defined, 14
    responsibilities of, 22
Surrogacy
    gestational, 100
    law and, 100

Termination of parental rights
    court hearing for, 105–106
    court hearing in, 105–106
    legal standard for, 105
    petition for, 104–105
Termination of services, limitations of, 61–62
Testamentary capacity, test of, 79–80
Testator, capacity of, to sign a will, 79–80
Testimony
    of child witness, 173, 174
    compelled, 48
    deposition, 174–175
    hypnotically induced, 186–187
    statutory criteria for, 78
    subpoened, 48–49
    testator, 77–78
    of witnesses, 77–78, 173–175
Third-party payer, 24. *See also* Insurance reimbursement
    defrauding, 30
    disclosure of information by, 50
Trademark infringement
    civil liability for, 211

ABOUT THE AUTHORS

Bruce D. Sales, PhD, JD, is professor of psychology, sociology, psychiatry, and law at the University of Arizona, where he also directs its Psychology, Policy, and Law Program. Among his other works are *Experts in Court: Reconciling Law, Science, and Professional Knowledge* (with D. Shuman); *More Than the Law: Behavioral and Social Facts in Legal Decision Making* (with P. English); *Courtroom Modifications for Child Witnesses: Forensic Evaluations* (with S. Hall, in press); *Family Mediation: Facts, Myths, and Future Prospects* (with C. Beck); *Treating Adult and Juvenile Offenders With Special Needs* (coedited with J. Ashford & W. Reid); *Ethics in Research With Human Participants* (coedited with S. Folkman); *Doing Legal Research: A Guide for Social Scientists and Mental Health Professionals* (with R. Morris & D. Shuman); *Law, Mental Health, and Mental Disorder* (coedited with D. Shuman); and *Mental Health and Law: Research, Policy and Services* (coedited with S. Shah). Professor Sales, the first editor of the journals *Law and Human Behavior* and *Psychology, Public Policy, and Law,* is a fellow of the American Psychological Association and the American Psychological Society, and an elected member of the American Law Institute. He received the Award for Distinguished Professional Contributions to Public Service from the American Psychological Association, the Award for Distinguished Contributions to Psychology and Law from the American Psychology–Law Society, and an honorary Doctor of Science degree from the City University of New York for being the "founding father of forensic psychology as an academic discipline."

Michael Owen Miller, JD, PhD, is a judge of the Superior Court in Pima County, Arizona. Judge Miller is the author of numerous articles on trial practice, mental health law, and juvenile delinquency. He also is the coeditor (with B. Sales) of a national book series on laws affecting mental health professionals. The series is based on *Law and Mental Health Professionals: Ari-*

zona that was coauthored by Judge Miller. Before his appointment to the bench, Judge Miller was in the private practice of law for 17 years, particularly focusing on litigation and administrative law in the areas of medical product liability and health care law. He was a principal participant in rewriting Arizona law to move it from psychologist certification to licensure. Judge Miller has also been very active in legal ethics and discipline, including chairing the committee that substantially revised the ethical rules for Arizona attorneys. More recently, Judge Miller was able to return to the Juvenile Court, which is the point where he began his law–psychology career more than 30 years earlier as the court psychologist.

Susan R. Hall, JD, PhD, is an assistant professor of psychology at Pepperdine University, Graduate School of Education and Psychology. During her postdoctoral fellowship in child clinical psychology at the Yale University School of Medicine, Child Study Center, she also was a Bush Fellow at the Yale Center for Child Development and Social Policy. Professor Hall has published and presented nationally on topics related to psychology, public policy, and law, such as legal issues in psychotherapy and child witnesses. Accordingly, her research and her new book *Courtroom Modifications for Child Witnesses: Forensic Evaluations* (with B. Sales, in press) examine the forensic assessment of children and youth exposed to violence and maltreatment. Professor Hall serves on the editorial board of the *Journal of Youth and Adolescence,* and she is a member of many professional organizations, including the American Psychological Association, American Psychological Society, American Bar Association, American Psychology–Law Society, Christian Association for Psychological Studies, and American Professional Society on the Abuse of Children.